D1605827

EEG IN CLINICAL PRACTICE

Second Edition

EEG IN CLINICAL PRACTICE

Second Edition

John R. Hughes, M.D., Ph.D., D.M. (Oxon.)
Professor of Neurology
Director of Clinical Neurophysiology
Director of Epilepsy Clinic
University of Illinois
College of Medicine at the Medical Center
Chicago, Illinois

Butterworth-Heinemann
Boston   London   Oxford   Singapore   Sydney   Toronto   Wellington

Every effort has been made to ensure that the drug dosage schedules within this text are accurate and conform to standards
accepted at time of publication. However, as treatment recom-
mendations vary in the light of continuing research and clinical
experience, the reader is advised to verify drug dosage schedules
herein with information found on product information sheets.
This is especially true in cases of new or infrequently used drugs.

∞ Recognizing the importance of preserving what has been
written, it is the policy of Butterworth-Heinemann to have the
books it publishes printed on acid-free paper, and we exert our
best efforts to that end.

Library of Congress Cataloging-in-Publication Data

Hughes, John R., 1928–
    EEG in clinical practice / John R. Hughes. — 2nd ed.
      p.   cm.
    Includes bibliographical references and index.
    ISBN 0-7506-9511-0 (alk. paper)
    1. Electroencephalography. I. Title.
    [DNLM: 1. Electroencephalography. WL 150 H893e 1994]
RC386.6.E43H84 1994
616.1'207547—dc20
DNLM/DLC
for Library of Congress   93-48489
                                       CIP

British Cataloguing-in-Publication Data.

A catalogue record for this book is available from the British
Library.

Butterworth-Heinemann
313 Washington Street
Newton, MA 02158

10 9 8 7 6 5

Printed in the United States of America

Contents

Preface to the Second Edition

For the past few years a number of readers have encouraged me to provide a new edition of this book. I delayed taking this action, since the theme of my book had been the basic principles in EEG, which should not often change. As a result, this new edition is a compromise between an attempt to expand nearly all areas with new information, and a tendency to avoid an encyclopedic account that would destroy the major intended features of this book: its brevity and simplicity. I have achieved this compromise by adding some recently described patterns, new figures, and many new references. I hope that you, the reader, will be even more pleased with the second edition than you were, as indicated by your many kind comments, with the first edition.

Preface to the First Edition

After serving as a Professor of Neurology for many years, I decided to return to medical school as a student (again) and was disappointed with many of the medical texts. Not only was the subject matter complex, but more importantly many of the texts were difficult to understand. Only a few authors presented their material in a clear, simple way, as exemplified by an elementary text on electrocardiography (Dubin), requiring less than 2 hours to arrive at approximately the same level of understanding as reading one of the more classical texts that required 10 to 20 hours. At that time I decided to write a text on EEG with emphasis on simplicity and clarity. Many physicians (interns, residents, psychiatrists, pediatricians, internists, and neurologists) and medical students have asked me to recommend a book that easily summarizes EEG and does not assume a sophistication in the neurosciences. I have tried to write a text for all physicians, except the *full-time* (board-certified) professional electroencephalographer, and to explain simply the technique of EEG, the normal and abnormal rhythms, in addition to their correlations and significance. Since the referring physician receives the EEG report in terms of normal or abnormal patterns, I have organized the text in terms of these EEG patterns (and also in the more traditional way, according to disease entity). This approach seems simpler, especially because the EEG is often similar for a variety of clinical disorders of different etiology. In addition, this book was written for the many neurologists who have considerable contact with EEG, including interpreting records, but who are not and should not be satisfied with their training in EEG during their residency. With many thousands of EEG laboratories in the United States and only hundreds of board-certified electroencephalographers, the great majority of those interpreting EEGs have had only brief and inadequate training. It is important, however, to make clear that no book, including the present one, can convert an inadequately trained neurologist into an electroencephalographer with considerable expertise. On the other hand, this book was designed to fill in the gaps of knowledge for this large group of neurologists and also to provide a simple overview of EEG for all other interested physicians. Finally, experienced technicians should find this book very helpful if they are interested in learning more about EEG in general to help in bridging the gap between themselves and the electroencephalographer.

Certain references to the literature and also many *exceptions* to the general points made in the text are *excluded* for purposes of *simplification.* Many other books contain these details.

The section on pen deflection and polarity is more lengthy than might be expected and provides many illustrative examples. The reason for this treatment is that most electroencephalographers do *not* completely understand these points; hence, a more detailed treatment was considered necessary. In addition, considerable space is given to premature, neonatal, and infant EEG, since simple texts on this general topic are scarce and possibly nonexistent. Also, physicians are utilizing EEG more in these infants, as progress is made toward understanding the complex patterns recorded from these tiny patients. Other special topics include (1) recording in the intensive care unit since brain death has become such an important topic of the day and also (2) medicolegal EEG in view of the legalistic world in which we presently live. These latter chapters will likely be of greater interest to those actively engaged in EEG interpretation. Finally, there are a number of controversial waveforms that could be summarily dismissed as insignificant patterns. Some of them, however, are commonly noted and also some electroencephalographers of considerable experience believe that they may be or are significant. Therefore, a brief reference is made to some of these patterns.

CHAPTER 1

Technique

Basic Elements Needed for the Electroencephalogram (EEG)

For the recording of brain waves (the EEG) we need: (1) *electrodes* to pick up the electrical activity and their attached wire to connect with the EEG machines, (2) *amplifiers*, since these rhythms are only microvolts (millionths of volts) in amplitude, (3) *filters*, often expressed as time-constants, since very slow or very fast (artifactual) rhythms at times need filtering out, and (4) *writer units* to record these rhythms on paper, moving usually at 30 mm/sec (also 15 or 60 mm/sec).

Electrodes

Electrodes usually consist of a flat disc or cup (often gold or silver) connected to an insulated wire. Needle electrodes can be used on comatose patients and still in some laboratories are used on awake patients, but they can be painful and can carry (hepatitis) viruses.

Position of Electrodes

Although other systems ("Gibbsian," "Michigan," "Houston") have been used successfully in the past, the great majority of EEG labs throughout the world utilize the 10–20 International System of Electrode Placement[1] (each electrode is 10 or 20 percent away from a neighboring electrode). Electrodes have identifying names: those on the left side have odd numbers; those on the right, even; near the midline, smaller numbers; and more lateral, larger numbers. The name includes the first letter of the general area where the electrode is placed.

$F_p1,2$ = prefrontal   T3,4 = mid-temporal
F3,4 = frontal   T5,6 = posterior temporal
C3,4 = central   A1,2 = ear (or mastoid)

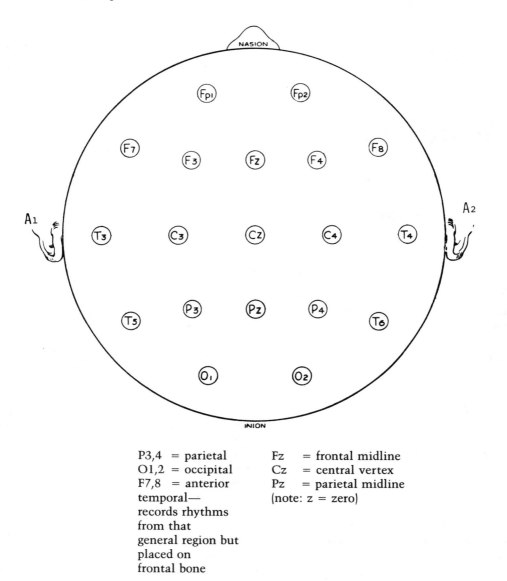

P3,4 = parietal
O1,2 = occipital
F7,8 = anterior
temporal—
records rhythms
from that
general region but
placed on
frontal bone

Fz   = frontal midline
Cz   = central vertex
Pz   = parietal midline
(note: z = zero)

International 10–20 system (measured)

Electrode positions are determined by measurements from different land-marks on the head.

(1) On the basis of 10 percent of the circumference of the head measured just above the eyebrows and ears, the position of the more peripheral electrodes is in part determined.

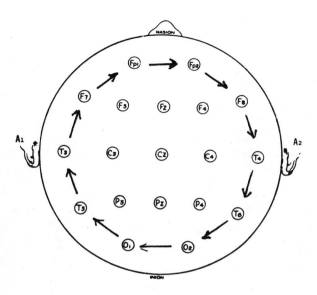

(2) On the basis of a measurement from the nasion to the inion, the position of the more central electrodes is in part determined.

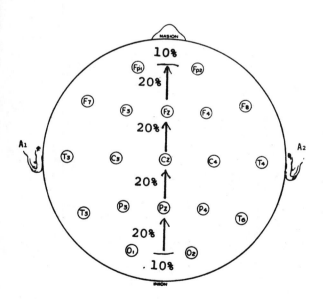

(3) On the basis of the measurement from the small fossa just anterior to the ear canal over the central vertex to the opposite side, the position of the coronal electrodes is in part determined.

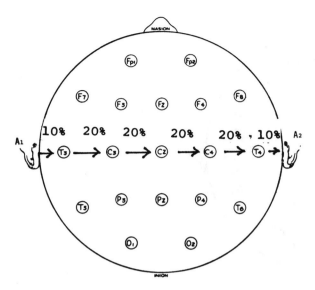

(4) The frontal electrodes are halfway between (1) the prefrontals and centrals and (2) anterior temporals and frontal midline and the parietal electrodes are halfway between (1) the centrals and occipitals and (2) posterior temporals and parietal midline.

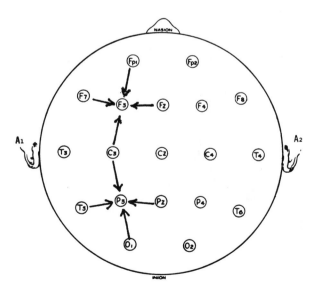

The determination of electrode position by these latter measurements is highly recommended; however, under certain (*emergency*) conditions these positions may be estimated.

International 10–20 system (estimated)

X = electrode position being determined
● = electrode position previously determined

Note that nose is down in these figures.
(1) Prefrontals (F_p1, F_p2) = 1″ (25 mm) above middle of eyebrow.

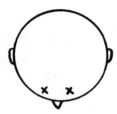

(2) Mid-temporals (T3, T4) = 25 mm above fossa anterior to ear canal.

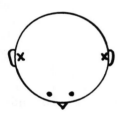

(3) Occipitals (O1, O2) = 25 mm above and lateral to inion.

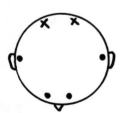

(4) Anterior temporals (F7, F8) = midway between prefrontals and mid-temporals on a circumferential line around the head.

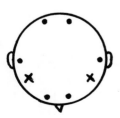

(5) Posterior temporals (T5, T6) = midway between mid-temporals and occipitals on a line around the head.

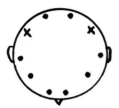

(6) Central vertex (Cz) = middle and top of head on a line from the mid-temporals.

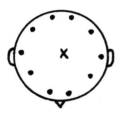

(7) Centrals (C3, C4) = midway between central vertex (Cz) and mid-temporals (T3,4).

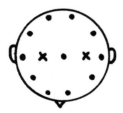

(8) Parietals (P3,4) = midway between centrals (C3,4) and occipitals (O1,2).

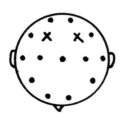

(9) Frontals (F3,4) = midway between centrals (C3,4) and prefrontals (F_p1,2).

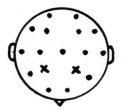

(10) Frontal midline (Fz) = midway between frontals (F3,4) and on the midline; parietal midline (Pz) = between parietals (P3,4) and on the midline.

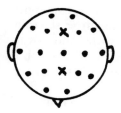

(11) Ears (A1, A2) = behind each ear lobe on the mastoid.

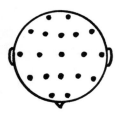

(12) A "ground" electrode is also added often on the mid-forehead, but it can be placed anywhere on the head or body. This electrode helps to eliminate 60 cycle interference that may be recorded as artifact.

Electrode Application

Electrode positions are now determined, and these areas are cleaned with acetone. Electrode paste is applied both to hold them in place and to improve the conductivity between the scalp and the electrode. Cotton or gauze often is placed over the electrode and its cream to help hold everything in place. Collodion (liquid) is sometimes applied onto the gauze placed over the electrode and is then dried by a jet of air. Electrodes secured by this means are usually firmly in place and do not easily loosen. For certain recordings, such as 24-hour ambulatory monitoring, the collodion technique for securing electrodes is mandatory.

Connections to EEG Machine

Each electrode has a wire (or lead) connected to it that gets plugged into an electrode board and conducts the electrical activity from the head to a particular designated connection on that board. From the board a large cable conducts the activity from each of the electrodes to the EEG machine.

Electroencephalograph (EEG Machine)

Elements

The EEG machine consists of 8 to 24 (or more) separate channels, each with its preamplifier, filtering circuit, and power amplifier, leading into a separate writing unit. The recommended number of channels is 16 to 18, and in various small offices or hospitals, using EEG not for precise localization but only as a screening device, 8 to 10 channels are often used. Under no circumstances, however, should fewer than 8 channels be used.[2]

The EEG machine utilizes the differential amplifier, as symbolized below:

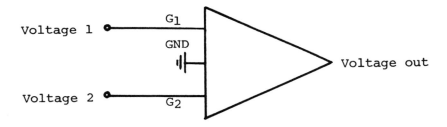

G_1 is input 1 with its voltage 1 (V_1) and G_2 is input 2 with its voltage 2 (V_2). Voltage out will be proportional to the *difference* between V_1 and V_2. If $V_1 = V_2$, then there will be no difference and no voltage out. If $V_1 = 10\mu V$ and $V_2 = 0$, this difference will be $10\mu V$; if the voltage out $= 10V$, the *amplification factor* can be determined and will be:

$$\frac{10V \text{ (out)}}{10\mu V \text{ (in)}} = \frac{10,000,000\mu V}{10\mu V} = 1,000,000$$

Unwanted signals, like 60 cycle interference from the "mains," which are in-phase (changing exactly in the same direction) as applied to both input 1 and input 2, should be canceled in this differential amplifier since the output is proportional to the *difference* between V_1 and V_2. How well this rejection is accomplished is given by the term *common mode rejection* (CMR), expressed in terms of a ratio, such as 5000:1, meaning that the unwanted signal at the electrodes (G_1 and G_2) will have its amplitude decreased by a factor of 5000 at the level of the pen write-out. This value is determined by connecting a voltage source between (1) the interconnected G_1 and G_2 inputs and (2) ground and comparing the output when the same voltage source is between (1) only one input and (2) ground. When G_1 and G_2 are interconnected, the output will be low, such as 1, and when they are not interconnected, the output will be high, for example, 5000, yielding a CMR of 5000:1.

Most EEG machines have a 60 cycle "notch" filter to eliminate any artifact from the "mains" that was not rejected by the CMR; also, other filters are used to eliminate activity under, for example, 0.5, 1, or 5 c/sec and above 15, 35, and 70 c/sec. Standard EEG is run usually with the low filter on 1 (or 0.5) and the high filter on 70.

Calibration

Calibration is an operation to determine if each channel properly responds to unidirectional pulses (50 μV), positive and negative, as seen in Figure 1.1. A channel with pulses too high or too low can be adjusted to the proper height by dials, sometimes called "equalizers." This latter calibration is performed without any patient in the system so another test is then done *with* the patient connected to the recording system, usually designated as "patient calibration." A short tracing is run with each channel recording exactly the same activity (often $F_p1 - O_1$) so all channels should look alike, as seen in Figure 1.2.

Montages

The EEG really consists of recording the brain's electrical *potential*, accomplished by recording the *difference* between the activity picked up by *two* electrodes. Montage refers to the different ways to connect electrodes; usually, two kinds are used: (1) referential (previously called "monopolar") and (2) bipolar.

Referential (Monopolar)

Referential recording involves the difference between an *active* electrode on the scalp (called "scalp electrode") and an *inactive* electrode, usually placed away from the scalp, for example, on the ear, nose, or chin (called "indifferent" or "reference electrode"). Often the indifferent electrode will be on the ear and, since it is still close to the temporal lobe, will pick up some brain

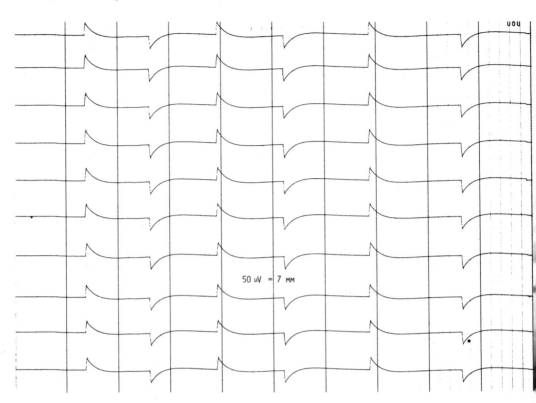

FIGURE 1.1   Calibration of the EEG machine. Pulses directed up and down are shown fo each of the 10 channels: each waveform should look the same since the same electrical signa is presented to each channel. The amount of signal is 50 microvolts (μV) and the deflectio measures 7mm in height, so each millimeter in height represents approximately 7 μV in volt age ($\frac{50}{7}$ = 7.1 μV/mm).

wave activity and therefore will not really be indifferent (only relatively in-different). The old designation *mono*polar is a poor term since it implies that one can record from one pole (or one electrode), but two poles or elec-trodes are required to record potential difference. Indifferent electrodes on the chin or nose (or anywhere else on the body) have a disadvantage in that they usually pick up a great deal of activity from the heart and therefore include these rhythms as artifacts into the recording.

Bipolar

The other of the two ways to record the EEG is called bipolar and involves the *difference* between two *active* scalp electrodes. Each *channel* of the EEG machine is connected to two different *electrodes*, and the *difference* in activity picked up by each of those two electrodes is recorded on that one channel.

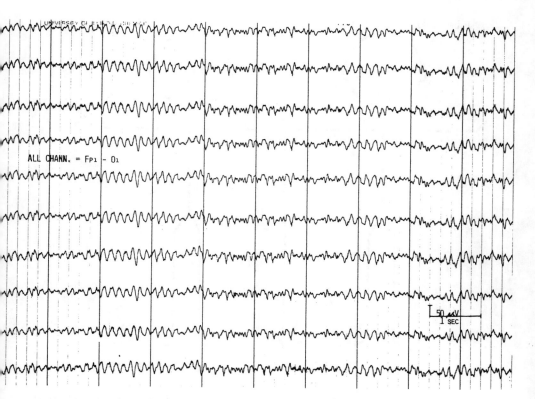

ALL CHANN. = Fp_1 - O_1

50 µV
1 SEC

IGURE 1.2   Patient calibration. Now the patient is included in the recording and each chan-
el is recording the same linkage of electrode Fp1 to O_1; thus, each channel should look the
ame as all others. On this and the following EEG samples, note the time calibration (length
f horizontal line representing 1 second in time) and voltage calibration (length of vertical line
epresenting 50 µV in voltage).

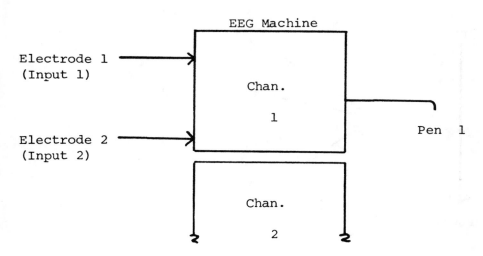

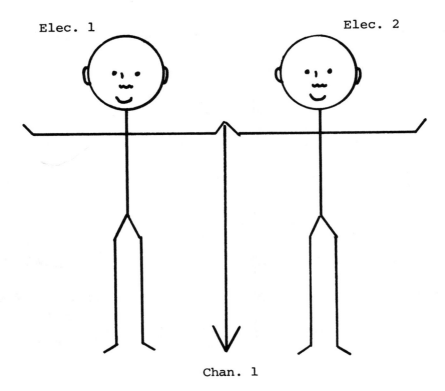

Chan. 1

Another way to represent two electrodes contributing to one channel: Montages (also called runs) should be arranged in an orderly sequence, often with the anteriorly placed electrodes on the first channels and the posteriorly placed electrodes on the latter channels.

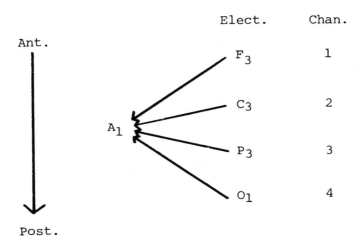

This run would be a referential montage with all left-sided electrodes referred to the same ear (left)–A_1 electrode. Arrows are used to designate each channel, recording from one electrode to another. The other four channels of an eight-channel machine would properly be the right-sided electrodes referred to the right ear–A_2 electrode.

Chan.   Elect.

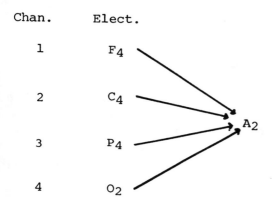

Another way to organize the montage is to alternate left- and right-sided electrodes from a general region so that a comparison is made between the two frontal areas (left and right), then the two central regions (left and right), etc.

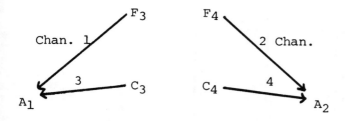

Bipolar montages are also arranged in an orderly way in chains, usually front to back or side to side, from one electrode to its neighbor and then onto the next one, etc.

Each channel has input 1 and 2 from the two electrodes connected to it, and arrows are again used to designate each channel, recording *from* one electrode *to* another. Note that C_4 electrode provides input 2 of Channel 1 and also input 1 of Channel 2. Electrode P_4 is the input 2 of Channel 2 and and input 1 of Channel 3, etc. Also, note that both F_4 and C_4 contribute to Channel 1. As schematized on the next page, the "movement of the arm" of either electrode can change the output of that channel.

Further details regarding technique, especially guidelines for standards, have been published by the American EEG Society.[2]

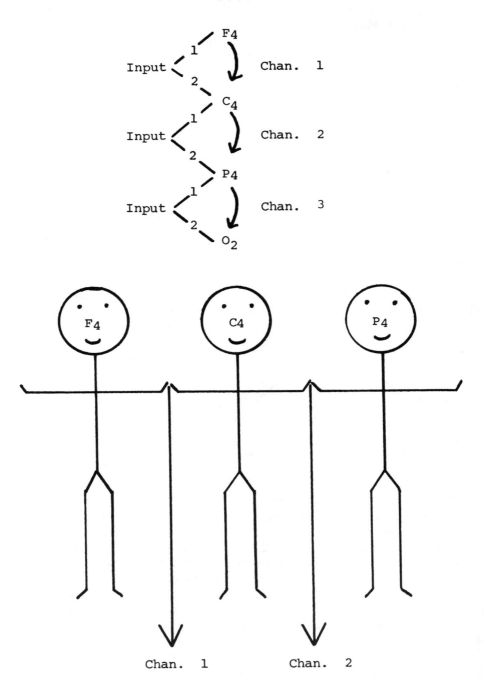

CHAPTER 2

Names of Rhythms or Patterns

Major Frequency Ranges of Rhythms

Electrical activity from the brain consists primarily of rhythms, and these rhythms are named according to their frequency in cycles per second (c/sec), also called Hertz (Hz):

- Delta refers to all rhythms less than 4 c/sec
- Theta is between 4 and < 8 c/sec
- Alpha is between 8 and 13 c/sec
- Beta is > 13 c/sec

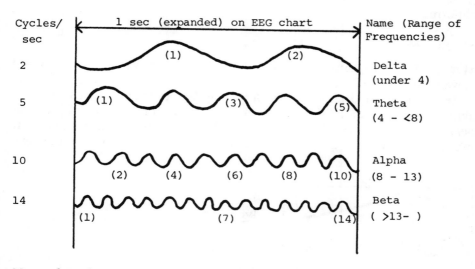

Normal Background Rhythms—Introduction

These different rhythms are found at different ages of the patient and also under different conditions. Usually, there is one dominant frequency, one that is the most prominent or obvious in the record, and this is called the "background rhythm."

1. Background rhythm in wake:
    in infants = 4 to 5 c/sec (Delta and Theta waves)
    in children = 5 to 8 c/sec (Theta)
    in adults = 8 to 10 c/sec (Alpha)
2. Background rhythm in sleep:
    in light sleep = 5 to 6 c/sec (Theta)
    in deep sleep = 2 to 3 c/sec (Delta)

Background rhythm can be considered as a general indication of the excitability of the central nervous system. It speeds up with increasing age (to adulthood) and slows down in sleep, especially with deeper sleep. Beta waves (faster than 13/sec) are normally seen in three conditions, especially on the frontal and central areas: (1) in light sleep in the form of 14/sec "spindles" = suddenly appearing and disappearing ᷧᷧᷧᷧ; (2) in tense and anxious patients at 15 to 20/sec frequency; (3) in patients on certain drugs that have a depressant action on the brain, especially the barbiturates and benzodiazepines at 18 to 25/sec in frequency.

Abnormal Patterns—Introduction

Abnormal patterns are mainly divided into two types: (1) slow waves and (2) spikes (or sharp waves). Also, depression of normal rhythms may be abnormal.

Slow waves

Slow waves are rhythms, appearing especially during wakefulness, that are slower than in the normal. Thus, an adult should not have theta or delta patterns in the waking record and if they appear, they are called slow wave abnormalities. Usually, the slower the frequency and the more often it appears, the greater is the degree of abnormality. Abnormal slow waves appear when the brain cells are damaged regardless of the cause of the damage.

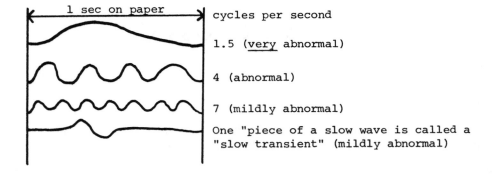

1 sec on paper	cycles per second
	1.5 (<u>very</u> abnormal)
	4 (abnormal)
	7 (mildly abnormal)
	One "piece of a slow wave is called a "slow transient" (mildly abnormal)

Paroxysms: spikes (sharp waves)

The spike (or sharp wave) is a suddenly appearing (paroxysmal) electrical explosion that looks on the paper record like a spike or large nail.

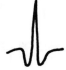

The sharp wave is the same as a spike, except for a difference in the duration of the event. Spikes are shorter in duration, usually <70 msec (approximately 1/14 of a second), while sharp waves last from 70 to 200 msec (1/14 to 1/5 of a second).

These two related patterns usually signify an epileptogenic region of the brain and are found in patients with seizures.

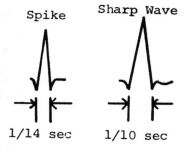

Another pattern related to the spike is the spike and wave complex, which consists of a spike followed by a wave. These complexes usually repeat themselves, especially at the frequency of 3/sec and at times under 3/sec or at 6/sec when bilateral.

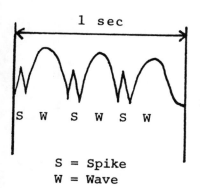

3/sec spike and wave complex

Depression of normal rhythms

One other form of abnormality in EEG is the depression (decreased amplitude) of any normal rhythms. These depressions can be seen during wake or sleep.

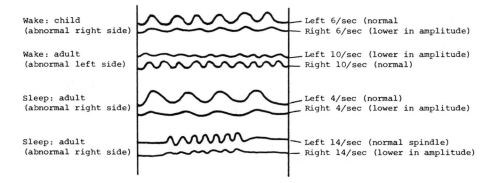

Wake: child
(abnormal right side)
— Left 6/sec (normal
— Right 6/sec (lower in amplitude)

Wake: adult
(abnormal left side)
— Left 10/sec (lower in amplitude)
— Right 10/sec (normal)

Sleep: adult
(abnormal right side)
— Left 4/sec (normal)
— Right 4/sec (lower in amplitude)

Sleep: adult
(abnormal right side)
— Left 14/sec (normal spindle)
— Right 14/sec (lower in amplitude)

CHAPTER 3

Localization Techniques

Referential Recording

The major responsibility of the electroencephalographer interpreting the EEG is to recognize the presence of abnormal patterns (slow waves or spikes), but also to localize them to a certain area of the brain. In referential recording (monopolar) this is accomplished by simply noting the electrode that records the highest amplitude of that abnormal pattern. All abnormal patterns usually spread out over a few electrodes and do not simply appear on only one, just as a stone landing in a pond makes a large ripple where it lands, but the ripple spreads out all around the point of entry. The electroencephalographer determines where the abnormal pattern is maximal and that is then the area of the brain with the neurophysiological disturbance.

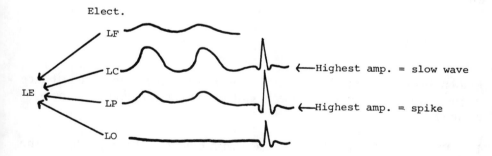

This example is a referential recording with left-sided scalp electrodes referred to the ipsilateral (left) ear (LE). The slow waves are seen on the left frontal (LF), left central (LC), and left parietal (LP) areas, but are clearly maximal on the LC area, the area of the brain with the disturbance. The spike is highest in amplitude on the LP area, the region producing this event, which also spreads out over other regions and appears on the LC and LO areas.

19

Bipolar Recording

*Bi*polar refers to *two* "poles" or two active electrodes from which we record. In this case the electrodes will be on the scalp (not the ears) and the linkage of electrodes for each montage will usually start at the front and run consecutively in a chain to the back of the head

Example:

F   frontal

↓

C   central

↓

P   parietal

↓

O   occipital

or at one side and run in a chain to the other side.

Example:

LE ——→ LT ——→ LC ——→ C ——→ RC ——→ RT ——→ RE
ear   temp.   cent.   mid.   cent.   temp.   ear
                         cent.

    Left   Right

Bipolar recording is a technique used for localizing the maximal disturbance in the brain, and this technique is called *phase reversal.* The important principles are:

1. Phase reversal is a technique used with bipolar recording to locate the area of maximal EEG abnormality.
2. The linkage of electrodes for the different recording channels must *run into* the abnormal area and then *run out of* that area.
3. Abnormal waveforms on the EEG will then appear on two adjacent channels and the pens will show deflections in opposite directions to each other, that is, they will show a "phase *reversal.*" A negativity on a given electrode causes the pens to come together and a positivity produces a separation.

4.   The electrode common to the two adjacent channels with the phase reversal sits over the brain area with the abnormality.
5.   EEG abnormality under electrodes that only begin or end an electrode linkage will not show phase reversal with that linkage since the montage does not run *into* and also *out of* the area. The channel with the electrode *beginning or ending* a linkage will show deflections in the same direction (in-phase) as neighboring channels, all pointing *up* to the electrode beginning the run or pointing *down* to the one ending the run in the case of a negative sharp wave.

Summary   In bipolar recording look for two adjacent channels with opposite or reversed phases; the electrode common to those channels gives the localization of abnormality. Electrodes beginning or ending a run show abnormality with the same phase in adjacent channels, pointing up to the electrode beginning the montage and pointing down to the electrode ending the run with negative sharp waves.

Let us illustrate bipolar recording using the example shown earlier with referential recording. The montage will begin on the LF area and run in a chain to the LO area.

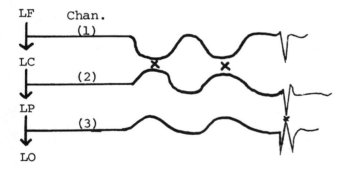

Each channel of the EEG must record between two electrodes. Channel 1 records from the LF to the LC area, Channel 2 from the LC to the LP, and Channel 3 from the LP to the LO area. The slow wave is seen reversing between Channels 1 and 2. The electrode common to those two channels is the LC and is therefore the electrode with the maximal slow wave abnormality. The spike is seen reversing between Channels 2 and 3. The electrode common to those two channels is the LP, and is therefore the electrode with the spike abnormality. The difference in the way to localize the maximal abnormality by referential and bipolar recordings can be viewed as follows.

Imagine the surface of the head as a flat surface with a mound representing the area of abnormality:

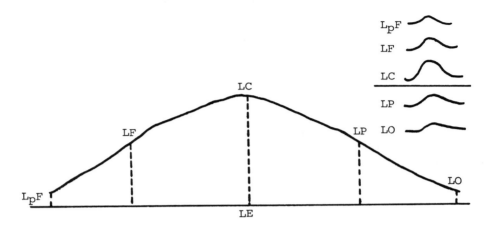

The reference electrode (LE = left ear) is represented at the surface of the head and the amount of abnormality is greater at LC than at the other areas. Since *differences* are recorded between the activity at two electrode locations, the difference between LC and LE is the greatest of five electrodes and is therefore the localization of the abnormality (see upper right).

In bipolar recording, close attention must be paid to which electrode is input 1 and which is input 2 on each channel of the montage (see below right).

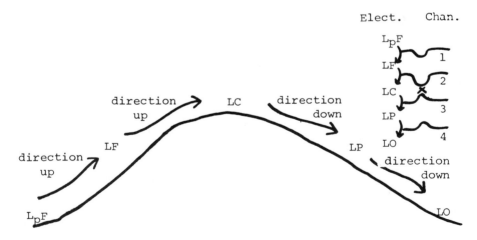

In Channel 1, the recording is *from* L_pF *to* LF (note the direction of the arrow in the linkage on the right diagram) and the abnormality is higher on LF than L$_p$F. In Channel 2, the recording is *from* LF *to* LC and again the abnormality is higher on the second of the two electrodes, namely LC. *But*, in Channel 3, recording *from* LC *to* LP, now the abnormality is *lower* on the second electrode of the pair and the trend is *reversed*. This is another way to think of phase reversal, as a way to localize the maximal abnormality. Look for the electrode in which the linkage up to that point shows one direction of change and beyond which then shows the opposite or reversed change.

Phase and Direction of Pen Deflection

In referential recording, the pens representing activity from different electrodes all move in the *same* direction up and down ("in-phase") to demonstrate the abnormality. In bipolar recording a phase *reversal* occurs on the two adjacent channels that have the common electrode with the maximal abnormality. When a phase reversal occurs, it is important to understand why each pen goes up or down. One way to understand why each pen goes up or down is to *memorize* the following convention used in all EEG machines.

positive ⟶ Negative   =   pen dowN

negative ⟶ Positive   =   pen uP

This designation means that a channel, recording from a positive electrode *to* a negative electrode, will send its pen down and a channel, recording from a negative (input 1) to a positive electrode (input 2), will send its pen up. A mnemonic aid is to remember that the first letter of input 2 is the last letter of the direction of change

$$\left(\text{Pos} \xrightarrow{\text{to}} \text{Neg} = \text{down}; \text{Neg} \xrightarrow{\text{to}} \text{Pos} = \text{u}p\right).$$

Here negative and positive refer to the polarity (direction) of the electrical activity or to whether the electrical force is above or below an electrical zero point, including how much above or below that point. This introduces the important point that polarity on a given electrode is *relative* with regard to its paired electrode. Thus, the *absolute* polarity of a waveform from two electrodes is not significant, that is, whether both are negative or both are positive; it is only the *difference* between the two that counts—which one has *relatively more* negativity and which one has *relatively more* positivity.

One way to understand this point is to view polarity as a value, positive or negative, on a continuous scale above or below a zero (0) point.

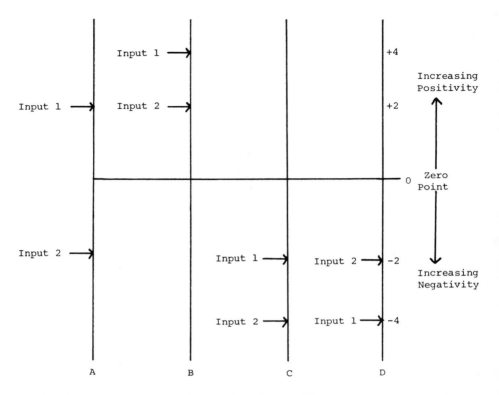

In this diagram an input *"above"* the other will be designated relatively *positive* (and an input below will be negative). Note in A, B, and C that input 1 is "above" input 2 and therefore more positive. Hence:

A, B, C: input 1 ⟶ input 2

(pos) ⟶ (<u>n</u>eg)   =   pen dow<u>n</u>

The pen will go down in all three instances even though both inputs in B are positive (above zero) and both in C are negative (below zero). In D input 1 is "below" input 2 and therefore more negative. Hence:

D: input 1 ⟶ input 2

(neg) ⟶ (Pos)   =   pen uP

The pen in D will go up, therefore, even though both inputs are negative.

Given the conditions, what will the pattern be?

Focus *Within* a Given Linkage These simple principles can be applied to the localization of *any* kind of activity (normal or abnormal), but the example of a sharp wave or spike discharge as recorded on a referential montage provides a simple example and is now presented. In the following examples negative values are assigned to electrodes with spikes because most spikes or sharp waves are primarily negative in polarity. Also, this negativity spreads out around the highest point, the focus, and does not restrict itself only to the focus.

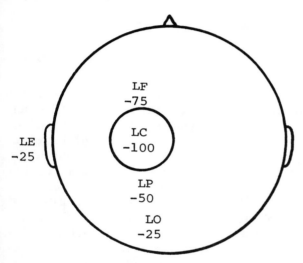

Assume a spike discharge located directly under the left central area (LC), consisting of −100 (negative) units. Since each abnormality spreads out over neighboring areas (like ripples from a stone thrown into a lake), the spike will be seen elsewhere too. On the left frontal area (LF) −75 units may be seen, on the left parietal (LP) −50 units, and on the left ear (LE) and left occipital area (LO) −25 units. In this referential recording each scalp electrode is referred to the ear. Hence:

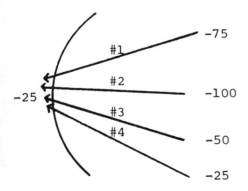

The numbers 1 to 4 indicate the four channels that will record this activity, and the arrows show input 1 (with values varying from −25 to −100) *to* input 2 (−25).

Chan.	Input 1	Input 2	Difference	Deflection	
#1	−75	−25	50	⋀	(up)
#2	−100	−25	75	⋀	(up)
#3	−50	−25	25	⌒	(up)
#4	−25	−25	0	—	(no change)

Since it is the *differences* between input 1 and 2 that are recorded, the greatest difference (75) is found on Channel 2, the next greatest (50) on Channel 1, the next (25) on Channel 3, and no difference is found on Channel 4, which looks at two electrodes with the same (−25) value and therefore without any difference between them. Note that the LE (input 2) electrode does have a value other than 0 and will frequently record brain waves, mainly from the temporal area, and therefore is not absolutely an "indifferent" electrode. The recording of the Channels 1, 2, and 3 will be negative → positive since −75, −100, and −50 are all more negative than −25, and all three pens will go up (negative → positive = up). Thus, Channel 2 will be the highest and Channel 1 (LF area) will go up more than 3 (LP area) since 50 units of difference are greater than 25. Channel 4 will show no change since no *difference* is noted between inputs 1 and 2.

As in all referential recordings the localization of this spike would be on Channel 2 from the left central (C3) electrode by noting that it has the *highest amplitude.*

Let us look at this same example on a bipolar montage.

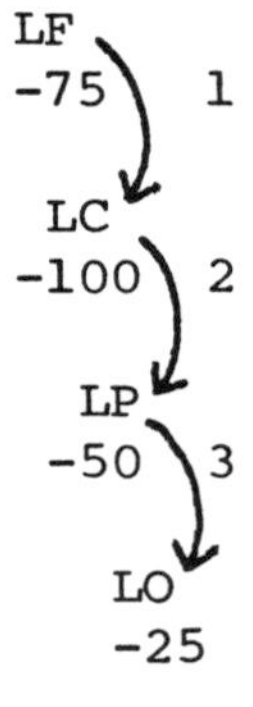

LF
−75   1
LC
−100   2
LP
−50   3
LO
−25

The montage with the chain of electrodes will be:

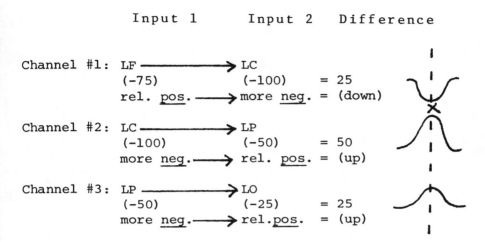

        Input 1   Input 2   Difference

Channel #1: LF ⟶ LC
             (-75)   (-100)   = 25
             rel. <u>pos</u>. ⟶ more <u>neg</u>. = (down)

Channel #2: LC ⟶ LP
             (-100)   (-50)   = 50
             more <u>neg</u>. ⟶ rel. <u>pos</u>. = (up)

Channel #3: LP ⟶ LO
             (-50)   (-25)   = 25
             more <u>neg</u>. ⟶ rel.<u>pos</u>. = (up)

In Channel 1, although both inputs are negative, −100 is more negative than −75 (which is therefore *relatively* positive) and so the input 1 → 2 is positive → negative (pen down). In Channel 2, −100 is more negative than −50, so input 1 → 2 is negative → positive (pen up) and a reversal will be seen between Channels 1 and 2. In Channel 3, −50 is more negative than −25, so 1 → 2 is negative → positive (pen up). Note that the phase reversal is seen between Channels 1 and 2 and the common electrode, namely the left central (LC), is the area with the maximal abnormality. Note also that the amount of deflection in Channel 2 is twice that of Channels 1 and 3 since the *difference* on Channel 2 was twice that on the other channels. Everything said about these spikes and their appearance on referential and bipolar montages is also true of slow waves, but examples of spikes are easier to present since they have primarily one phase (deflection), rather than alternating up and down, as with slow waves. Slow waves are localized exactly the same way as spikes by determining (1) the highest amplitude on a referential (monopolar) montage and (2) a phase reversal on a bipolar montage.

Focus at the *Beginning* of a Linkage If a focus exists at the beginning of a linkage, then a phase reversal *cannot* be seen (see Principle 5) since the run does not come into and also out of this area. With the same montage just used, an example is now given of a spike discharge on the LF area, the first electrode at the beginning of a montage.

Note that input 1 is more negative than input 2 (negative → positive) in all three channels, so they will all go up (in-phase) and there will be no phase reversal. The up-deflection *points to* the left frontal area where the spike is localized.

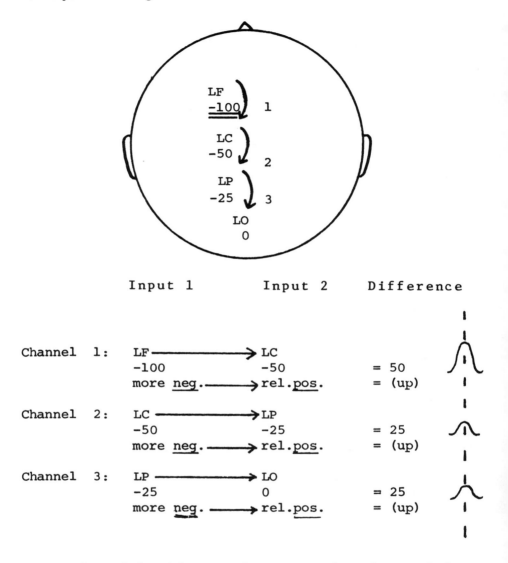

Focus at the *End* of a Linkage   In the same way that a focus at the beginning of a run cannot show a phase reversal, a focus at the *end* of a run cannot, since the montage does not run into and out of that area. An example
of a spike discharge on an electrode at the *end* of the same bipolar linkage
is now given.

In Channels 1, 2, and 3 the deflection will be down since input 1 is each
time relatively positive and input 2 negative. Thus, all three channels will
go down, as if pointing to the left occipital area where the spike discharge is
actually located. No phase reversal will appear since the linkage ends on the

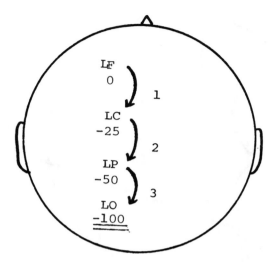

	Input 1	Input 2	Difference	
Channel 1:	LF ⟶ LC			
	0	-25	25	
	rel.pos. ⟶ more neg.		(down)	
Channel 2:	LC ⟶ LP			
	-25	-50	25	
	rel.pos. ⟶ more neg.		(down)	
Channel 3:	LP ⟶ LO			
	-50	-100	50	
	rel.pos. ⟶ more neg.		(down)	

area with the abnormality, and therefore there can be no common electrode on adjacent channels for a reversal.

A Positive Focus An interesting situation pertains in the case of a phenomenon called 6 to 7 and 14/sec positive spikes seen maximal on the posterior temporal areas ($_pT$). In this case the spikes are primarily positive (an exception to the usual rule that the *major* polarity of most spikes is negative). The values under each electrode represent typical amplitudes, as are found with these positive spikes.

In Channels 1, 2, and 3 input 2 is always more positive than input 1 (which is more negative), so the pens will go u*p* (neg → *po*s). Note that Channel 2

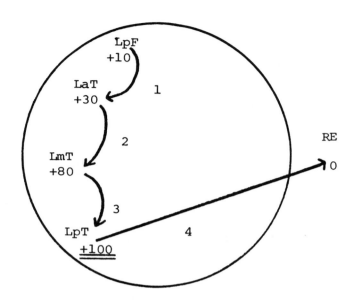

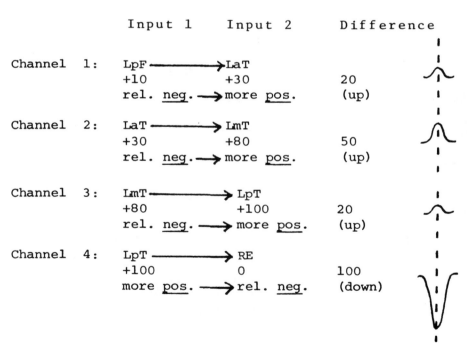

has a greater up deflection because the difference is 50 units, compared to 20 in Channels 1 and 3. Channel 4 shows a large down deflection (pos → neg). Thus, positive spikes go up in Channels 1 to 3 and down in 4. Note that a phase reversal does occur between Channels 3 and 4 since the L_pT electrode is the common electrode of the two channels best recording the spike. The reversal is not the usual "coming together" of the two pens, reflecting a primary negativity on the common electrode, but a "going apart" of those two pens, reflecting a primary positivity for that common electrode, as seen below:

PHASE REVERSAL

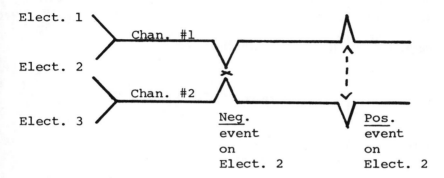

Brain rhythms recorded on an EEG machine follow the rules set down and illustrated in the last few sections. Each deflection, up or down, in each channel should be consistent with those few simple rules and all deflections should be internally consistent, one with the other. If not internally consistent, then usually that deflection is from an artifact, which refers to any recorded disturbance other than a brain rhythm. An example of a deflection *without* internal consistency is:

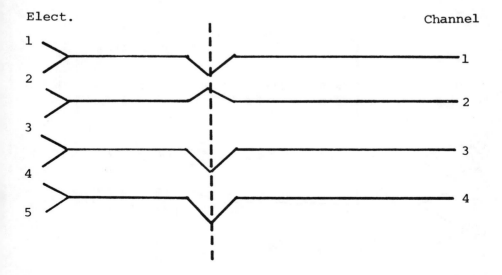

Channels 1 and 2 are coming together, reflecting a negativity on the common electrode 2, and Channels 2 and 3 are going apart, reflecting a positivity on the common electrode 3. Although theoretically possible, a negativity on electrode 2 with a simultaneous positivity on electrode 3 does not often occur in EEG and usually indicates artifact. Only rarely does the EEG show a (non-artifactual) simultaneous negativity and positivity in the form of a dipole (2 poles). When such a dipole appears, it is mainly seen with negative sharp waves on the central area and positive ones on the frontal area (as in Rolandic epilepsy, also known as centro-temporal epilepsy or benign epilepsy of childhood).

Given the pattern, what are the conditions?

With the simple rule:

(Input 1)   (Input 2)

negative ————————→positive = up deflection
positive ————————→negative = down deflection

the localization of *any* focus with *any* montage can be determined. For example:

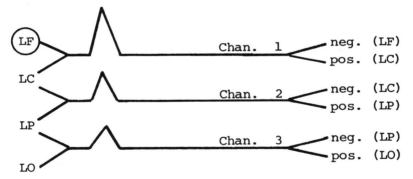

All three channels are going u*p* (neg → *pos*), without a phase reversal, as if pointing to the most anterior electrode, LF, where the focus appears.
    Another example of a focus is:

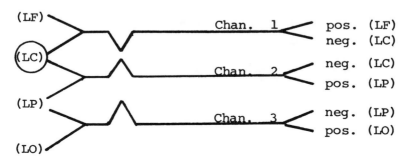

In Channels 1 and 2 the pens are coming together (pos → *neg; neg* → pos),
reflecting a major negativity or focus on electrode LC.

Another example of a focus is:

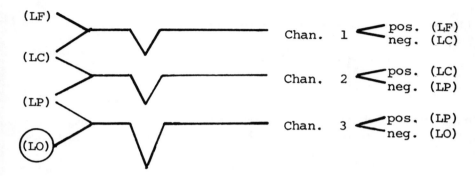

```
                              Chan.  1  <pos. (LF)
                                         neg. (LC)

                              Chan.  2  <pos. (LC)
                                         neg. (LP)

                              Chan.  3  <pos. (LP)
                                         neg. (LO)
```

All three channels show a down deflection representing positive → negative
in each electrode pair, pointing down to the main negativity on the LO area
where the focus is found. No phase reversal is noted since there is no common electrode with the focus that involves adjacent channels.

A phase reversal would be seen if we extend the montage to include an
electrode (for example) on the neck, as follows:

Electrode:

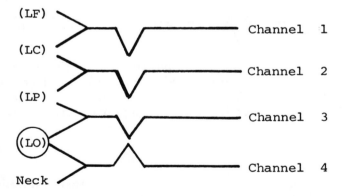

```
                              Channel  1

                              Channel  2

                              Channel  3

                              Channel  4
```

Now the LO electrode is the common electrode with a focus involving two
adjacent channels and the montage runs into that area (LP → LO) and out of
the same area (LO → Neck), so a phase reversal does occur.

Examples on a referential montage are simple to demonstrate:

Electrode:

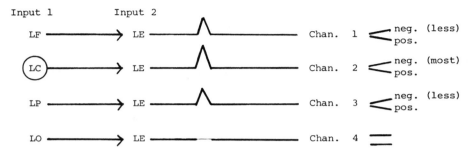

On the first three channels up-deflections are seen, all reflecting negative →
positive, and the focus is identified simply by looking for the highest negativity (Channel 2 on the LC area).

Since the ear electrode is in proximity to the temporal area and picks
up activity from that region, spikes from the temporal area often appear on
the ear electrode. On a referential montage this will appear as follows:

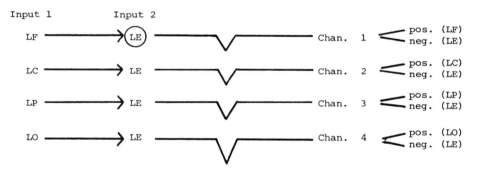

All channels will go down, each reflecting a positive → negative polarity
and indicating that the common electrode to all channels (the LE electrode)
has the negative focus. Since the left ear electrode is common to all four
channels as input 2, then the deflection should be approximately the same
size in each channel.

Equipotentiality

At times a focus spreads equally over two electrodes, rather than primarily
involving only one, and in this instance the two electrodes have an *equal
potential* on each. The area covered by the two electrodes is then an area of
equipotentiality. An example is shown below with hypothetical values:

Channel 2 shows almost a straight line, since the two electrodes contributing to it have the same (equipotential) value and therefore there is no difference between them. Channels 1 and 3 show a phase reversal (coming

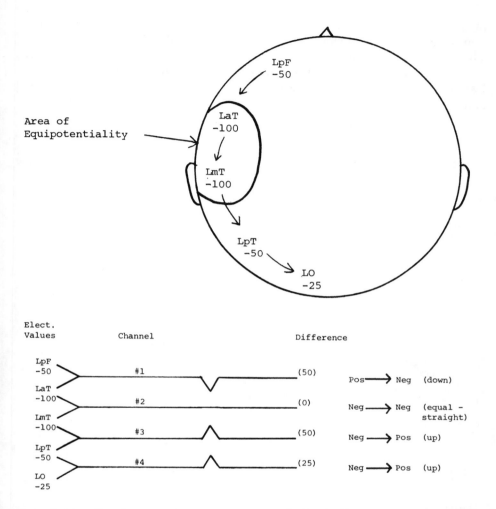

together), reflecting a major negativity, not from a given electrode, but from the *two* equipotential electrodes (LaT and LmT).

The following example illustrates the important points that (1) small deflections do not necessarily mean low amplitudes in a bipolar recording and also that (2) activity on a given channel may be coming from one or *the other* electrode contributing to that channel. The slow waves seen on the first three channels throughout the right side of the head are also seen on the last channel, which records the difference between electrodes Cz and LmT. One temptation would be to hypothesize that this right-sided slowing has been transmitted to the *left* temporal LmT electrode and for this reason appears on the last channel, 8. This interpretation would be incorrect. The slowing on the last channel is coming from the other of the pair of electrodes (Cz) as it spreads from the right side to the central vertex region. The

nearly flat Channel 7 does not represent inactivity but instead an equipotential region between the large area between the RmT and Cz electrodes.
Thus, the small or absent deflections on Channel 7 are not the result of
low amplitude or absent activity, and the high amplitude deflections on the
last channel are not from the LmT electrode but from the other one of the
pair, Cz.

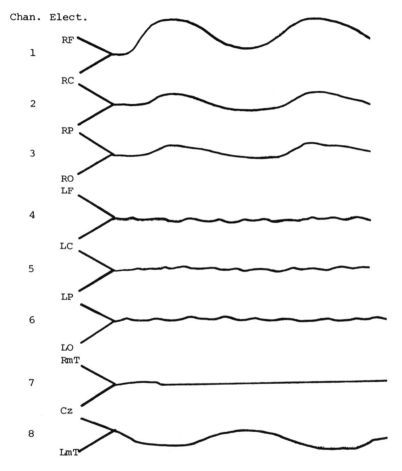

In assessing the *amplitude* of various rhythms, for example, the alpha,
referential recording leads to a more accurate assessment than bipolar
recording, which may, in fact, be misleading. This example illustrates
the point:

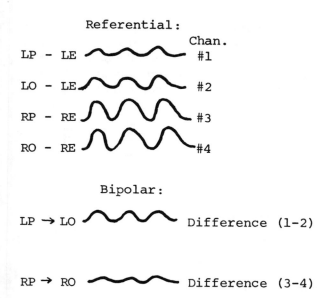

Referential:

LP - LE ~~~~ Chan. #1

LO - LE ~~~~ #2

RP - RE ~~~~ #3

RO - RE ~~~~ #4

Bipolar:

LP → LO ~~~~ Difference (1-2)

RP → RO ~~~~ Difference (3-4)

In the referential recording, the activity from the LP and LO areas is depressed, compared to the right side. On bipolar recording, however, the opposite *seems* to appear, except that careful inspection of the referential recording shows a greater *difference* between the LP and LO activity than on the right side. Thus, larger deflections appear on the left, when recording *differences* in a bipolar arrangement, even though lower amplitudes really appear on that same side, as seen by the referential recording.

The type of montage for accurate localization

Usually, a laboratory has a certain number of montages that are used on each patient; these runs are already wired into the EEG machine and can be selected by turning the appropriate dial. One simple rule for devising the minimal requirements for a complete battery of runs is to incorporate each electrode at least once in an anterior–posterior direction and also in a coronal arrangement. Both referential and bipolar runs are important; the former, by pairing widely separated electrodes, are especially effective in obtaining an overall picture of the rhythms and also for detecting subtleties, mainly diffuse low amplitude patterns; the latter, bipolar, are useful for a simple determination of the localization of a focus. During the recording the technician can devise any other run that helps to determine the exact localization of a focus. The simple rule is to devise a montage that criss-crosses over that focus, referring to chains of electrodes running both in an anterior–posterior and a coronal direction over the focus. Then, with phase reversals, the exact localization can be determined in both directions. If a montage shows a reversal from a chain of electrodes in only one direction, then only a partial localization can be given. For example, assume a focus under the left parietal (P3) electrode, which would likely appear to some extent on the neighboring left posterior temporal (T5) electrode. If a montage incorporated only the temporal electrodes, then a reversal would appear on T5 since this electrode senses the abnormality better than any other one used in the montage. One may not yet assume, however, that the focus is best seen on T5.

Chan.

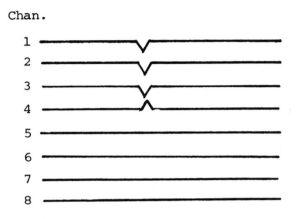

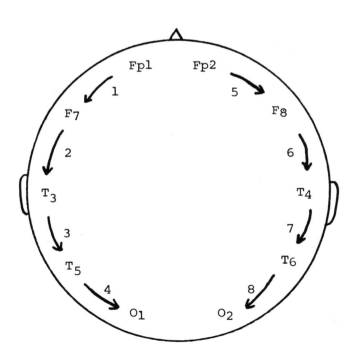

The next run to delineate the focus would be one using both anterior-posterior and coronal linkages:

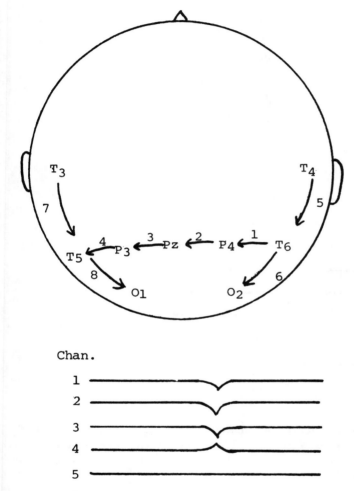

Now the reversal is seen between Channels 3 and 4, implicating P3 electrode, and between Channels 7 and 8, implicating T5 electrode. The first four channels show that P3 is more involved than T5 since the reversal is between Channels 3 and 4, with P3 as the common electrode. Since Channels 7 and 8 did not involve P3 and did record from T3, T5, and O1 and since

the reversal from the first four channels showed a maximal involvement on
P3, the run now to do is:

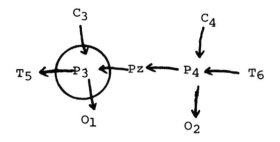

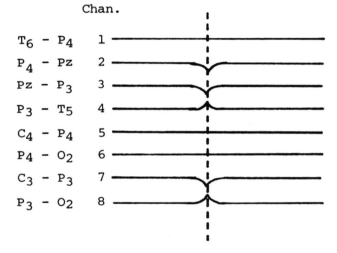

Now the focus has been clearly delineated in that P3 shows a reversal on
an A–P and also a coronal direction. The montage includes a criss-cross
of linkages over the area, showing a reversal in both A–P and coronal
directions.

CHAPTER 4

Artifacts

Muscle

Artifacts refer to any disturbance in the recording that does not arise from the brain. Since the EEG records microvolts (millionths of a volt), including the electrical activity from muscles under the scalp, the EEG often includes muscle *artifact*. This type of disturbance can appear as a single "blip," recognized usually as a muscle artifact by its very brief duration; as a series of blips at nearly *any* frequency; and finally as a burst of blips packed together at a very high frequency so that separate blips cannot be distinguished. See Figure 4.1 for examples.

60 Cycle

Artifacts can also arise from the 60 cycle power source. This artifact can be picked up by scalp electrodes, especially when these electrodes have a high electrical resistance from grease, dirt, or dead skin that must be cleaned from the scalp. One good rule is that a high resistance electrode picks up especially *all* kinds of artifact, not just the 60 cycle type. The resistance of each electrode connected to the different scalp areas is measured by an ohmmeter, and usually values of less than 5000 ohms are desired. The determination that an artifact in question is the 60 cycle variety can be made by recalling that it is exactly 60 cycles per second. Since EEGs are usually run at 30 millimeters (mm) per second (approximately 1⅛ inches per second) 60 deflections will be packed into the 30 mm space and will appear as a thick "dirty" line or possibly as crowded muscle activity. The difference between these two types of artifact can be clearly determined by running a brief segment of the EEG at fast speed (double the usual speed), 60 mm per second. Now the 60 deflections per second are not so packed since they have a 60 mm space to fit into and each individual regular deflection can now be counted and determined not as muscle artifact but as a 60 cycle distur-

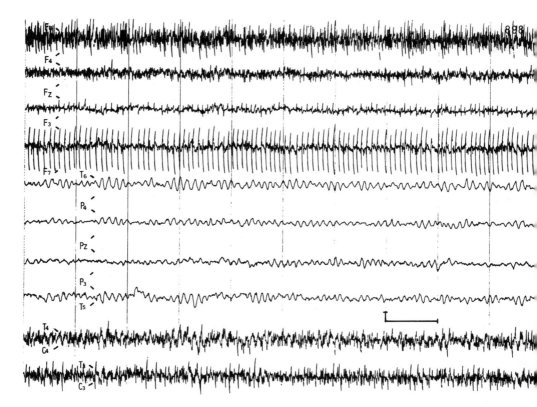

FIGURE 4.1   Muscle artifact. Contraction of muscles under the scalp results in this type c artifact, which can have an irregular, very spikey appearance, as seen on the Channels 1–2 9–10, or can appear as rhythmical sharp deflections, as noted on Channel 4 with any kind c frequency (here at 10/sec). Also, only a single deflection may be seen, rather than a series c these blips.

bance. In the case of muscle artifact, the deflections are not regular and not sinusoidal, but usually are irregular in frequency and amplitude (see Fig. 4.2)

Electrode Movement

Another type of artifact results when any electrode even slightly moves on the scalp. If the patient is lying down and the back of his head is on a pillow that is in contact with the O1 and O2 electrodes (occipitals), each time the patient breathes his head may go up and down, producing a slight rocking motion on those two electrodes. This rocking action of the electrodes may result in a movement artifact (see Fig. 4.3).

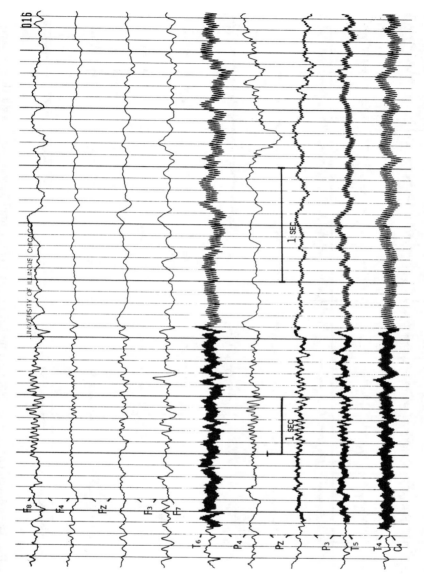

FIGURE 4.2   Sixty-cycle artifact. On the left the paper speed is the usual at 30 mm/sec, so the 60 cycle is so compact that it appears as a black line, but at the speed of 60mm/sec (on the right), each deflection can be counted and determined as 60 cycle artifact.

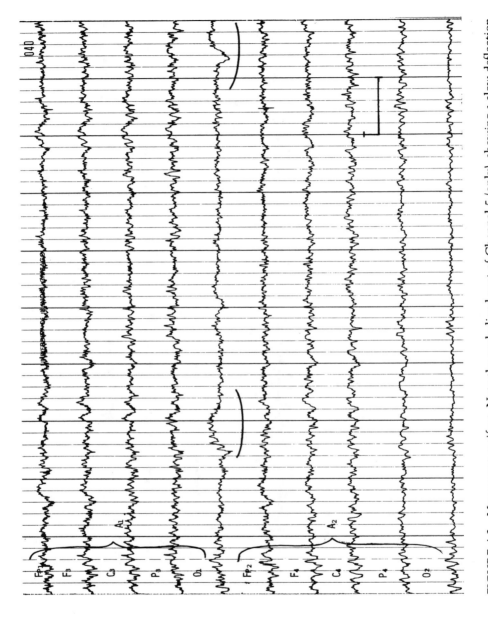

FIGURE 4.3　Movement artifact. Note the underlined part of Channel 5 (only), showing a slow deflection from movement of the head on the left occipital area.

Eye Movement

The eye is like a charged battery, with the positive (+) side on the corneal surface of the eye and the negative (−) side on the retina. This battery has a large voltage, so that when the eyes move they produce clear deflections on the EEG as "eye movement artifact." When a patient blinks a reflex (Bell's phenomenon) usually causes the eyes to go up as the lids close. Since the outside of the eyeball is charged +, this positivity is directed toward the nearest electrodes, Fp1 and Fp2, and makes them *more* positive than other neighboring electrodes. As the lids open, the eyes come down, moving away from Fp1 and Fp2 and producing a relative negativity on those electrodes. In a referential recording the following occurs.

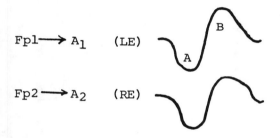

At A the lids close and the eyes go up, making Fp1 and Fp2 positive, so pos.→neg. (Fp1→A1, Fp2→A2) sends the pen down. At B the lids open and the eyes come down, making Fp1 and Fp2 negative, so neg.→pos. sends the pen up (at times overshooting) and then finally to the resting position (see Fig. 4.4). Lid movement is also important.

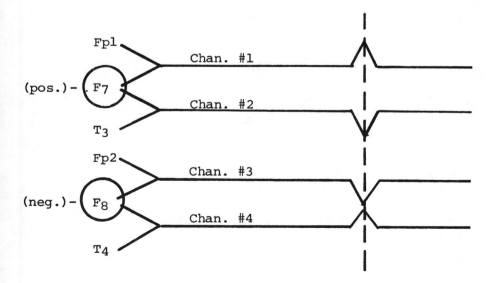

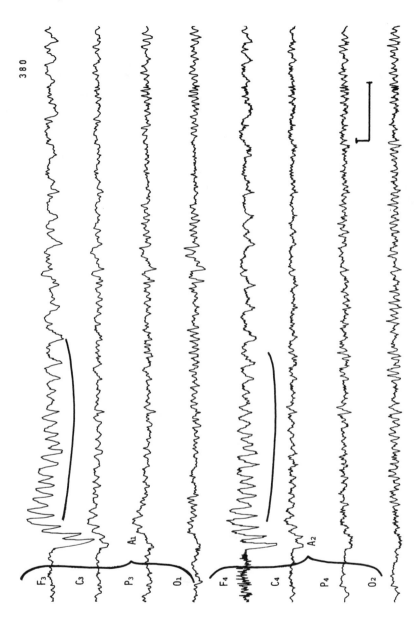

FIGURE 4.4   Eye flutter. Single eye-blinks are usually easily identified, but eye flutter at a fast frequency can often mimic slow waves on the frontal areas. Note Channels 1 and 5 showing 6/sec eye flutter, which is nearly as fast as this artifact can appear.

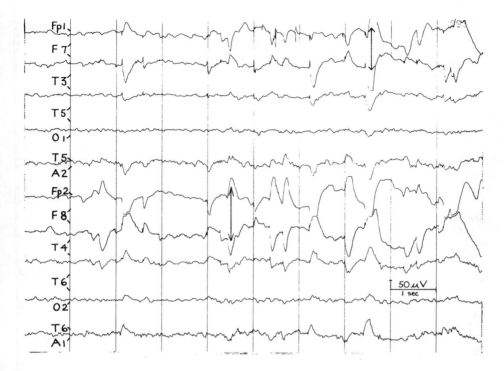

FIGURE 4.5   Rapid eye movements (REM). The montage is from the prefrontal, along the temporal, to the occipital areas with the top five channels on the left and bottom five on the right. The anterior temporal electrodes ($F_{7,8}$) are represented between Channels 1 and 2 and also 6 and 7, where rapid deflections are noted, representing the REM. When the pens separate, as seen at the first arrow between Channels 6 and 7, a positivity is reflected at that same moment when on the other side the pens come together, reflecting a negativity. The eyes are moving to the side where the positivity (pen separation) is noted (see arrow between Channels 1 and 2 when eyes are moving to the left).

Side-to-side movements of the eyes occur in which the positivity on the cornea comes closer to the F7 or F8 electrode making one of them positive, the one *toward* which the eyes are moving, and the opposite one negative, *from* which the eyes are moving. On the following montage a characteristic pattern is seen:

If the eyes are moving to the left, then the positivity on the cornea is directed to that left side (F7 electrode) and Fp1→F7 is neg.→*pos.* with an up-deflection on Channel 1. For the linkage F7→T3, a *pos.*→neg. will cause a down-deflection and the separation of the pens indicates clearly a *positivity* on F7. A negativity on F8 (since the positively charged cornea is *moving away* from F8) will cause the channel recording Fp2→F8 (pos.→*neg.*) to go

48   *Artifacts*

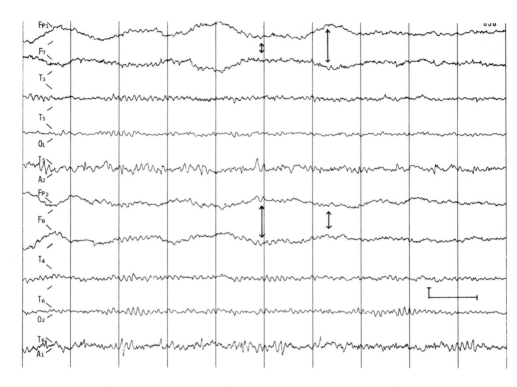

FIGURE 4.6   Slow eye movements (SEM). Note on Channels 1 and 2 from the left and 6 and 7 from the right, the very slow deflections, reflecting changes on the F_7 and F_8 electrodes. The eye, as a biological battery with positivity on the cornea, is moving to the right side at the first vertical arrow, inducing on electrode F_8 a relative positivity, seen as a phase reversal with a pen *separation*. At the same time an opposite phase reversal is seen on the other side (F_7) since the eyes are moving away from the left, creating a negativity on the F_7 electrode. At the second vertical arrow the eyes are moving slowly to the left (to the side of the positivity or pen separation).

down and the channel recording F8→T4(*neg.*→*pos.*) to go up. The pens on these latter two channels coming together indicate a corresponding relative *negativity* on that other side. The rule (on this run) is that eyes are moving toward the side where the pens *separate* (the *positivity*). Figure 4.5 shows an example of REM with side-to-side eye movements found in patients with narcolepsy with their sleep onset REM (SOREM) or in patients withdrawing from drugs affecting the central nervous system, especially alcohol. Slow eye movements (Fig. 4.6) represent an artifact similar to that from REM, except that they are simply slower, as the name implies. Rather than sudden, fast, jerky movements of the eyes, usually from side to side (REM), SEM refers to slow eye movements lasting up to 5–6 seconds in duration and also usually from side to side. They are often seen in (normal) afternoon sleep and therefore represent a normal artifactual pattern.

Electrode Pop

Sometimes electrodes become defective and "pop" during the recording. This phenomenon refers to a sudden deflection, like a little "spark" or "blip" from the electrode, either negative or positive, but usually the latter. The popping may be related to some impurity in the metal portion of the electrode or some kind of particle on the electrode that reacts with the metal to produce the blip (see Fig. 4.7).

Sweating

Sweating from the patient usually causes a very slow artifact. As the perspiration, a type of salt solution, emerges from under and around an electrode the resistance of that electrode likely is changing continuously and the perspiration also probably loosens the electrode. These and other related changes cause a very slow deflection that is most troublesome since it often masks the brain rhythms (see Fig. 4.8).

Vascular

The heart and its related vessels account for at least two types of artifact. Since the heart is a muscle and contracting muscles produce electrical changes, each heart beat is associated with well-known prominent deflections, the EKG. The EKG can, of course, be picked up nearly everywhere on the body and to some extent on the head, especially on the electrodes (A1 and A2), often called "EKG artifact." The other type of artifact associated with the vascular system is more associated with the pulse. In this case an electrode is situated near a vessel that pulsates with each beat, producing slight movements of the surrounding tissue with each surge of blood through it and also slightly moving the electrode with each beat. A movement type of artifact then appears synchronized with the pulse, especially when the patient's head is resting on a given area with its electrode pressed down onto a nearby vessel. Moving the electrode slightly off the pulsating vessel is sometimes required, but repositioning the head to avoid pressing a given electrode down onto a pulsating vessel may also resolve the problem (see Fig. 4.9).

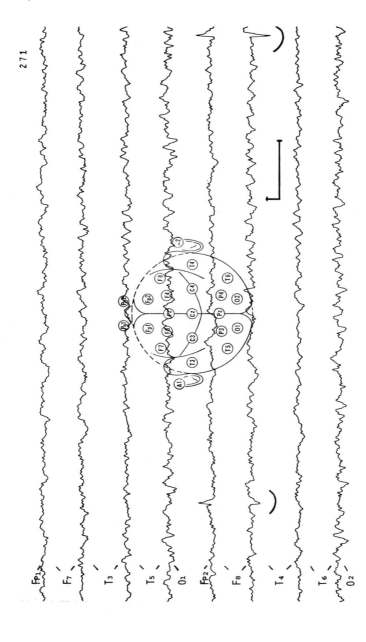

FIGURE 4.7 Electrode pop. Note Channels 5 and 6 (underlined) showing the pen separation (positivity) involving the popping electrode F_8.

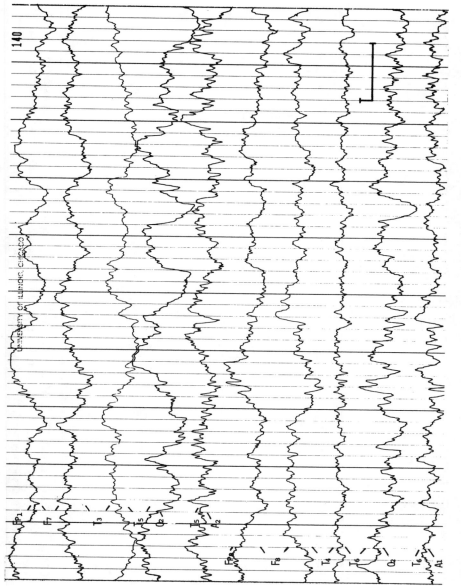

FIGURE 4.8   Sweat artifact. Note that high amplitude, slow irregular deflections appear on most channels, especially 1 and 2.

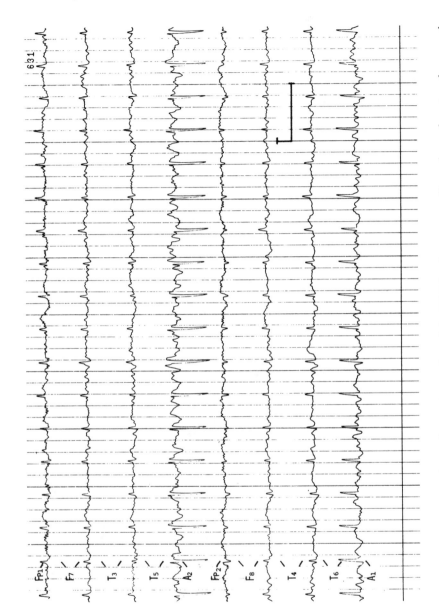

FIGURE 4.9   EKG artifact. The QRS complex of the EKG is often seen well on channels using the ear reference (see 4 and 8 here), but the sharp deflections can be seen on all channels. Pulse artifact refers to the slow deflections associated with the pulse, seen underlined in Figure 7.1C.

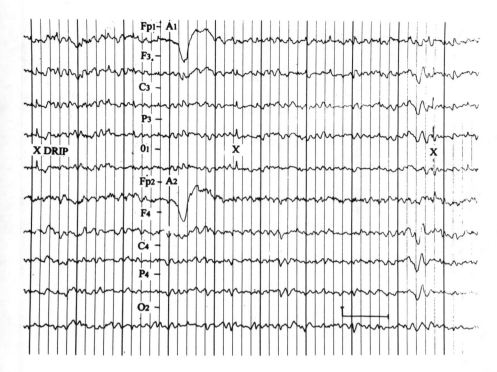

FIGURE 4.10 Drip artifact. Note the spike-like appearance of the drip artifact, appearing each time a drip in the IV line occurred. The first 5 channels are from the left side and last 5 from the right, all referred to the ipsilateral ear.

Other artifacts can certainly occur from broken wires, sudden voltage surges associated with nearby equipment, faulty elements within the EEG machine, and movements associated with respiration, sobbing, sucking, tremor, or swallowing.

Drip

The drip artifact can be seen on any or all channels of an EEG when there is a drip in a container of an intravenous line (Fig.4.10). Since these artifacts can appear very similar to a spike discharge, the EEG technician should indicate the timing of the drips with the appearance of the artifact for at least a part of the record.

CHAPTER 5

Normal Rhythms

State of Awareness

Waking

Locus

Earlier, a brief description was given of the waking EEG, but more details are given in this section. The alpha rhythm (8 to 13 c/sec) is the characteristic pattern seen in the waking record of normal adults, usually maximal on the occipital areas, but at times higher on the parietal areas. Not infrequently in the aged, the maximal amplitude appears anteriorly and may be found even on the frontal areas, called *rhythms of alpha frequency.*

Amplitude

The alpha is often equal in amplitude on the two sides (bilaterally symmetrical), but a slight decrease (<25%) of amplitude on the left is common. Since the alpha is the expression of the *resting* brain and the dominant hemisphere (the left side in right-handers) can be considered as the less "resting" or more "active," a *lower* amplitude of alpha may be expected from that hemisphere. Since the great majority (90% to 95%) of subjects or patients are right-handed with a left hemispheral dominance, the left side can be expected to show a lower amplitude of alpha, and frequently this difference does in fact appear. In approximately 50% of left-handers, the right side is dominant and in those relatively few individuals the right-sided alpha may be lower in amplitude. One good rule in EEG, however, is that a consistently decreased alpha amplitude on the right is often associated with an abnormality within that hemisphere,[3] while slight decreases on the left are usually normal. The association of alpha amplitude with hemispheral dominance has been controversial, because some investigators have found positive relationships[4] but others have not.[3] Nevertheless, a definite right-sided depression of alpha, as a 50% difference, must be considered suspicious as an abnormal finding, especially in a right-handed patient.

Synchrony

The alpha rhythm usually occurs at the same frequency on the two sides in a given phase relationship (bilaterally synchronous). A clear difference in alpha frequency between the two sides is extremely rare, and when it does seem to occur, often the slower frequency is really an *intermixed* high frequency theta (6.5 to 7.5 c/sec) rhythm rather than a low frequency alpha (8 to 8.5 c/sec) background rhythm.

Frequency

In the infant the background rhythm is often approximately 5 c/sec, maximal on the central areas.[5] In time a slight increase in frequency may occur, but soon the alpha waves (8 to 13 c/sec) also begin to appear and are maximal on the posterior regions and, by age 8 years, the background rhythm should be up to 8 c/sec.[3] The theta waves (4 to < 8 c/sec) characterizing the dominant rhythm on the central areas of the infants may remain while the alpha becomes more prominent posteriorly, and then the theta activity fades away and is usually gone by the late teens. During adulthood, a slight increase in the alpha frequency is often seen (from 8 to 10 c/sec).[3] In the older years the alpha frequency then decreases and frequencies below 8 c/sec are not uncommon after 65 yrs of age.[6] In the *healthy* aged, however, the mean frequency of the alpha remains above 8 c/sec, even in centenarians[7] (Fig. 5.1). Therefore, the "rule" is anyone of at least 8 years of age, including centenarians, should have an alpha background rhythm of at least 8 c/sec.

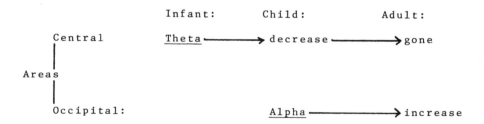

Sleep

Generally, the *slower* waves are associated with the *deeper* stages of sleep, but five distinct stages can be identified[8] (Fig. 5.2). The first, stage I (drowsiness), shows a decrease in the amplitude of the waking alpha so that no obvious rhythm is seen. The next, stage II (light sleep), shows symmetrical theta (4 to < 8 c/sec) rhythms, especially posteriorly, and vertex sharp transients and 14 c/sec spindles (the combination of the latter two events called *K-complex).* In stage III (moderately deep sleep), from 20% to 50% of the rhythms are symmetrical delta waves (under 4 c/sec) and in stage IV

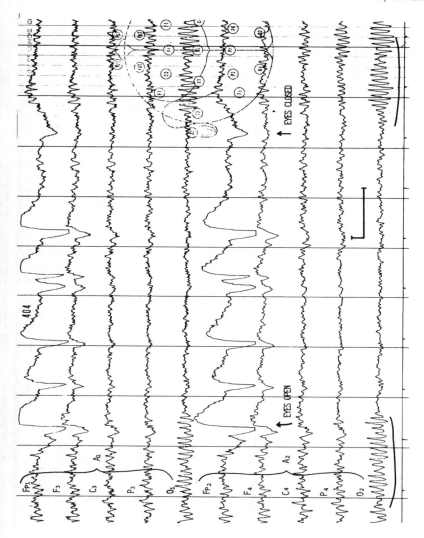

FIGURE 5.1   Alpha activity in resting adult. Note that the recording is a referential montage to the same ear with the first five channels on the left (front to back) and the last five on the right. The alpha is approximately 9½ cycles/sec, maximal on the occipital areas, disappears with eyes open, and reappears with eyes closed.

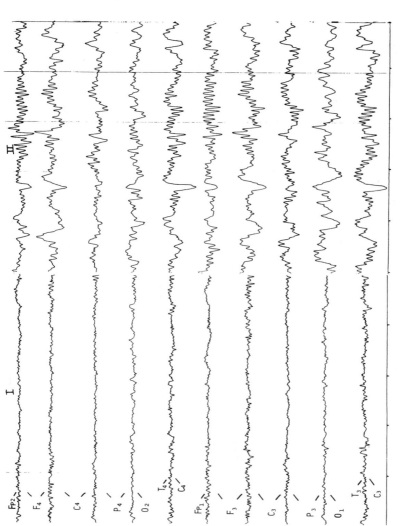

FIGURE 5.2   Sleep stages I through IV. On extreme left is stage I (drowsiness), showing low amplitude activity (loss of alpha); next is stage II, characterized by spindles and vertex sharp transients (K-complexes); followed by stage III, with 20% to 50% of the record with (symmetrical) diffuse slow waves under 4/sec; and on the extreme right is stage IV (deep sleep), with more than 50% of the record with diffuse delta rhythms. REM is the fifth stage (see Fig. 4.5). (See next page for continuation.)

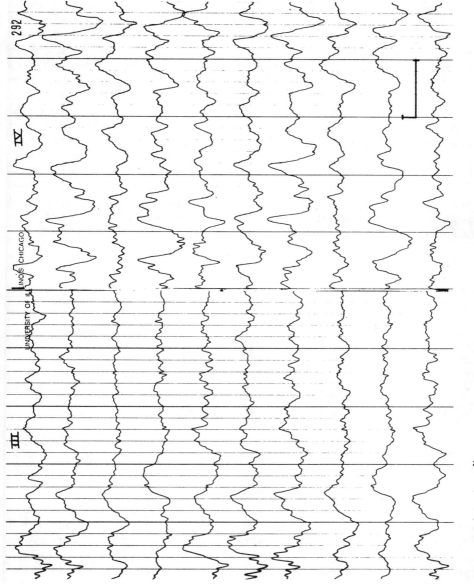

Figure 5.2 (continued)

(deepest sleep) over 50% are delta rhythms. The other remaining stage is the REM (rapid eye movement) stage (see Fig. 4.5). This is called REM because the eyes move quickly, especially from side to side. These different stages usually appear in an orderly manner as cycles throughout the night, and approximately four cycles appear each night. The REM stage in normals does not appear within the first cycle but waits for one complete cycle (stage I to IV and then back from IV to I) before appearing, usually 90 minutes after sleep onset. If REM does appear at first near the onset of sleep, this is called "early REM" and is usually seen in narcoleptics with other associated symptoms such as sleep paralysis (inability to move upon awakening), hypnagogic hallucinations (vivid visual patterns near sleep onset), or cataplexy (falling to the ground at the onset of an emotional experience).[9] Early REM is also seen in individuals withdrawing from depressants of the central nervous system such as barbiturates or alcohol.[10] The length of time in stage IV is greatest early during the sleep and then lessens later, and the REM stage is shortest at first and then lengthens later, especially near awakening.

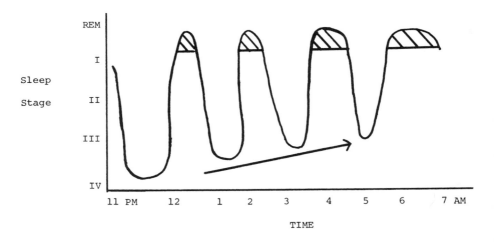

REM stage is often associated with dreaming, and if one awakens in the morning during a REM period, then that dream may be remembered. If one usually awakens at a time when some other stage is occurring (not REM), then dreams appearing at other REM stages earlier in the night usually will be forgotten. Thus, almost everyone dreams, but remembering the dream depends mainly on whether or not the awakening time coincides with a REM stage.

Activating Procedures

Hyperventilation

This procedure is used as an activation, especially of focal slow waves, but also of bilaterally synchronous spike and wave complexes of (corticoreticular) primary generalized epilepsy. Normal changes during hyperventilation (HV) are important to understand. These can be stated quite simply: any symmetrical slow waves appearing during HV are normal until proven otherwise.[3]

Waves as slow as delta rhythms are commonly found in younger patients, but also occasionally are seen in adults especially those who vigorously perform the HV to lower their pCO_2.[11] Rhythms of 2 to 3 c/sec, usually are seen diffusely, but are often maximal on the occipital areas in younger patients and on the frontal areas in older children or adolescents.[12] These delta waves may appear after theta rhythms have first been seen and the usual change during HV can be described as a gradual slowing of the background rhythm. Occasionally, these delta waves may suddenly appear as bursts, presenting a difficult interpretation as to whether they could be abnormal spike and wave (epileptic) patterns (with a hidden spike component), which also appear as sudden bursts. Without any clear spike component, the interpretation should be conservative: viz., they are a normal pattern as long as the slowing is relatively symmetrical. The difference in the child who *frequently* shows these very slow waves and the adult who *rarely* demonstrates these changes is likely related to two factors.[3] One factor is that the younger patients usually more vigorously perform the procedure and drive their pCO_2 down further than adults. The second factor is the evidence that the younger patients have more of a vascular or metabolic lability in response to pCO_2 changes. Although patients with other abnormalities in their EEGs more often show these slow wave changes (called "build-up" or "blow-up"), the presence of the slowing by itself should not be labeled abnormal, as long as the waves are symmetrical (Fig. 5.3).

Another important variable for a build-up during HV is a possible hypoglycemic condition, which predisposes the patient to show this slowing.[13] A child who has not eaten for a long period of time with delta waves during HV, who is then given orange juice or some other means of raising the blood sugar, will then later usually show less slowing during HV. This sequence of changes emphasizes that a metabolic factor seems involved in the production of diffuse slow waves associated with HV in children.

When a build-up occurs, further encouragement of the patient to continue the HV will not likely yield helpful data. If the response is diffuse delta waves at 2 to 3 c/sec, this effect is probably an appropriate end point and the patient should stop the HV. At times, the patient may develop a tetany based on changes of the binding of the calcium ion, and clinically the response may be viewed by the technician as "shivering."[14]

Photic Stimulation (see Figs. 5.4, 5.5).

Flashes of light are presented to the patient in 10-second periods at different frequencies (e.g., 1, 3, 6, 9, 12, 15, 18, and 24/sec). These stimulating frequencies will often "drive" the brain at the same frequency, a phenomenon called "photic driving," appearing maximal on the occipital areas. The

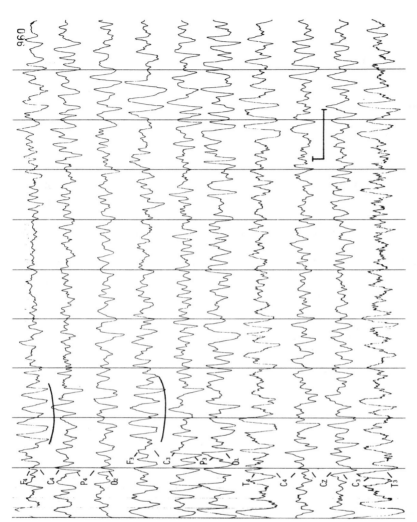

FIGURE 5.3   "Build-up" from hyperventilation (HV). Most bilaterally synchronous and symmetrical slow waves during HV should be considered normal. They are usually diffuse, but often appear maximal on the occipital areas in young children and on the frontal areas in older children.

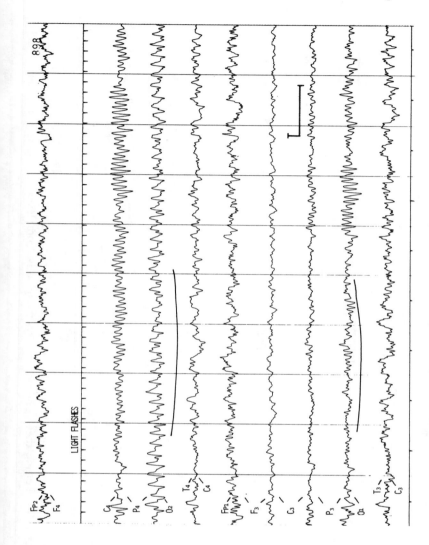

FIGURE 5.4 Photic responses depressed on one side. Channel 2 monitors the light flashes and Channels 4 and 9 show the responses to those flashes on the occipital areas (right and left, respectively). Note on the right (Channel 9) the decrease in amplitude of photic responses to each flash of the flickering light.

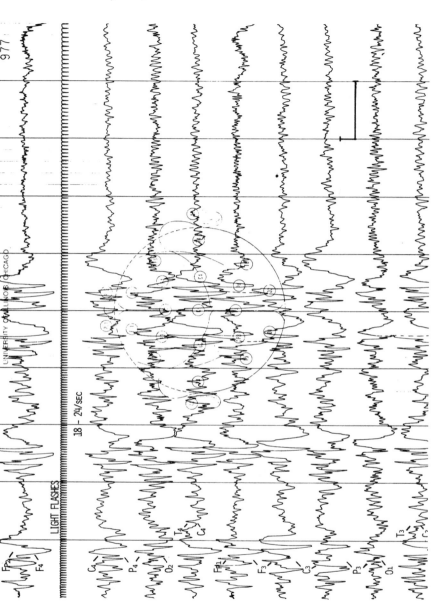

FIGURE 5.5   Photically elicited bilateral spike and wave complexes. Light flashes at 18 to 24/sec are usually more effective in eliciting these (epileptiform) spike and wave complexes than slower frequencies under 12/sec.

absence of any clear driving response, seen in approximately one-third of all patients,[15] does not constitute an abnormality nor does any rhythmical response at the fundamental, harmonic (double, triple, etc.), or subharmonic (one-half, one-quarter, etc.) frequency. An important variable in these photic responses is the amplitude, which should be equal (L. vs. R.) or within 25% of each other. A slight (<25%) depression on the left side is likely seen as frequently with photic driven responses as with alpha amplitude and is not only normal, but expected. A 50% difference with a left-sided depression, although not by itself abnormal, is suspicious of a left-sided abnormality and a 75% difference would likely reflect some organic change in that left hemisphere. As in the case of the alpha amplitude, a slight (25%) depression of photic responses on the right is usually more meaningful than on the left and a 50% change would likely be significant, indicating some abnormality within the right hemisphere. The one other reason to include photic stimulation as an activating procedure is to determine if bilateral spike and wave complexes can be elicited.

Sleep

THE NEED FOR A SLEEP RECORD IN ALL PATIENTS WITH A DEFINITE OR POSSIBLE SEIZURE DISORDER is emphasized more than once in this book. The confirmation of a seizure disorder will be found in the form of a spike or sharp wave discharge, often (about 80% of the time) appearing *only in a sleep tracing*. Therefore, if a *waking* record *only* is run on a patient with a possible seizure disorder and does not demonstrate a spike, the test should be considered incomplete, since the presence or absence of a discharging focus will not have been evaluated. Usually, sleep stages I and II, including spindles, are required (20 minutes) for an adequate sleep tracing to check on the possibility of a discharging focus. Rarely are stages III and IV of deep sleep required to demonstrate a sharp wave or spike focus.

Age

Premature

General Principles

The first important point to be made in this section is that correct interpretation of the EEG of premature infants depends on the knowledge of the gestational age (GA),[16] referring to the time from the first day of the last menstrual period to *birth*. THE MOST IMPORTANT VARIABLE, HOWEVER, IN DETERMINING THE EEG IS THE CONCEPTIONAL AGE (CA), defined as the GA *plus* the chronological age *after birth*. Thus, CA is time within the uterus plus time on earth after the birth.

The next important general principle is that the EEG develops the same whether the infant remains within the uterus or has been born and is living in the outside world.[17] Another way to make this point is to state that the EEG WILL BE SIMILAR FOR A GIVEN GA AS FOR THE SAME CA.

Another general principle in premature or neonatal EEG is that EEG ABNORMALITY IN THESE INFANTS MAY APPEAR ONLY IN THE FORM OF A PATTERN THAT IS CHARACTERISTIC OF A YOUNGER AGE THAN THE PATIENT'S STATED AGE.[18] These earlier patterns therefore reflect a neurophysiological immaturity of the brain (also called a dysmaturity) by demonstrating that the brain has not developed normally in its rhythms. In this section on premature infants, EEG examples are from babies a few days after birth and therefore GA will be used to designate age, since CA is then equivalent to GA.

Earliest Activity = Periods of Quiescence

The earliest EEG activity that can be recorded is at approximately 22 to 23 weeks of gestational age in those few premature infants that can survive long enough for an EEG recording at that age. The ACTIVITY AT THAT TIME IS NOT CONTINUOUS, BUT CONSISTS OF SHORT BURSTS INTERSPERSED AGAINST A FLAT OR QUIESCENT BACKGROUND[19] (Fig. 5.6). The bursting activity consists of slow (especially at 1/sec) and fast rhythms (especially at 10 to 14/sec).

The flat or quiescent periods, also called tracé discontinué, vary enormously in duration, and at the very early age of 22 to 24 weeks GA may vary from 5 sec to *8 minutes!* Thus, for a matter of minutes the EEG will show nothing but a flat recording until a short burst of activity interrupts the quiescence. The range of flat periods at 28 weeks is 10 to 40 seconds (Fig. 5.7) and at 30 weeks 3 to 10 sec (Fig. 5.8). Some data[20] are available suggesting that quiescent periods may also be seen beyond 34 weeks but other data argue that they no longer appear after 32 weeks, as indicated by the solid curve in Fig. 5.6.[21] The author's own data argue strongly for the former. Figure 5.9 shows some of these data,[22] indicating that *all* patients up to 32 weeks CA will show some quiescence (possibly only a few seconds), decreasing to 50% at 36 weeks, and only a few show this pattern near term. As quiescence tends to disappear, activity, of course, takes its place. The faster that quiescence is lost after 32 weeks, the more likely the premature infant will develop normally; the closer to term that quiescence continues to appear the more likely an abnormal development is expected. Statistically, clear quiescence at term can be considered abnormal and likely reflects a neurophysiological immaturity. If the quiescence represents more than 40% of the record anytime after 32 weeks, the prognosis is poor at 3 years of age. An additional note is that high levels of barbiturate medication can add to the amount of quiescence.

Quiescent periods must be differentiated from two other patterns, which can appear similar to them. A pattern called tracé alternant (see below and also Fig. 5.10) can look somewhat like the flat-burst combination of the premature, but the major difference is that *CLEAR ACTIVITY* CAN BE

PREMATURE EEG

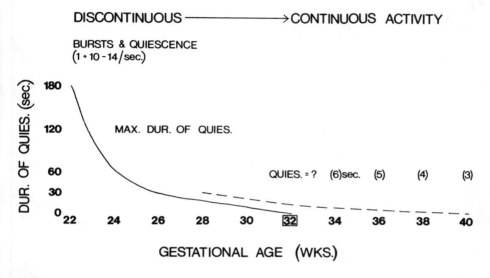

DISCONTINUOUS ——————————→CONTINUOUS ACTIVITY

BURSTS & QUIESCENCE
(1 ‧ 10 -14/sec.)

FIGURE 5.6 Earliest EEG activity in the premature, periods of quiescence and bursts of activity. Solid line shows the decrease in the longest duration of quiescence that can be seen at the different gestational ages up to 32 weeks, when continuous activity begins to appear. The dashed line shows the results of other data suggesting that quiet periods can continue until near term with (?) questionable periods of quiescence lasting 6 to 3 seconds from 34 to 40 weeks.

SEEN DURING THE DEPRESSED PORTION OF TRACÉ ALTERNANT,[17] IN CONTRAST TO *COMPLETE INACTIVITY* OR FLATNESS APPEARING IN THE EARLY PREMATURE INFANT. The other pattern that needs to be differentiated is a very abnormal one, called the suppression burst (Fig. 5.11), seen usually in pathological comatose states. In this case the differentiation is not made by checking the flat or depressed part of the record, as with tracé alternant, but instead by checking the bursts of activity. IN THE SUPPRESSION BURST RECORD OF A COMATOSE PATIENT, THE ACTIVITY TENDS TO BE *SHARPER* IN CONFIGURATION OR EVEN SPIKELIKE IN FORM, WITH MORE FREQUENCIES SEEN DIFFUSELY AT RELATIVELY HIGH AMPLITUDES.

Earliest Premature Patterns

Sharp theta on the occipitals of prematures (STOP) After quiescence, the earliest distinctive EEG pattern in premature infants is the STOP,[23] referring to 5 to 6 c/sec activity, sharp in configuration, either unilateral (53%) or bilateral (47%) in a given record and maximal on the occipital regions (see Fig. 5.12). Their incidence and amplitude are highest in the youngest of

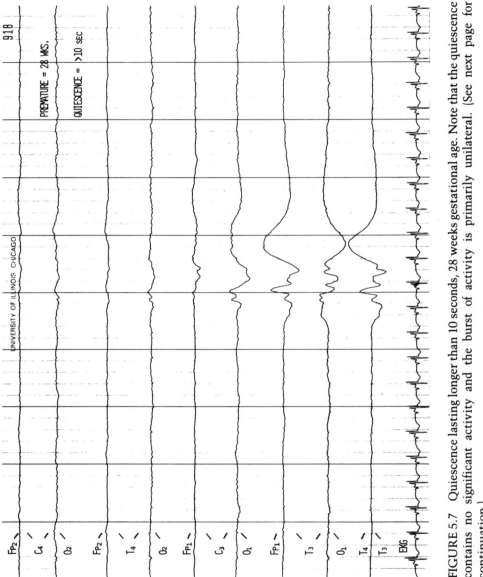

FIGURE 5.7 Quiescence lasting longer than 10 seconds, 28 weeks gestational age. Note that the quiescence contains no significant activity and the burst of activity is primarily unilateral. (See next page for continuation.)

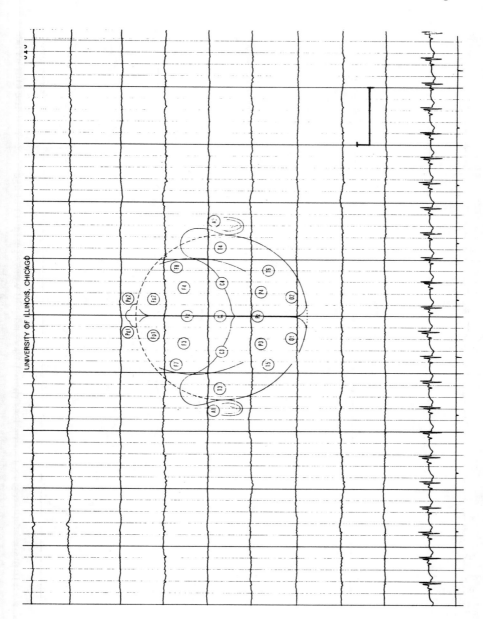

FIGURE 5.7 *(continued)*

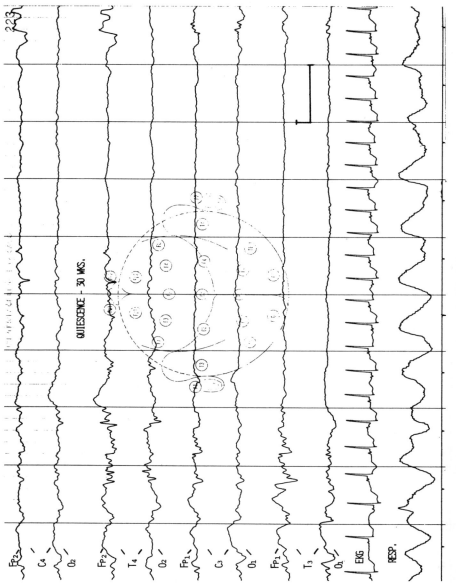

FIGURE 5.8   Quiescence lasting less than 10 seconds, 30 weeks gestational age. Note that the quiescence is seen first on the left side before appearing then on both sides.

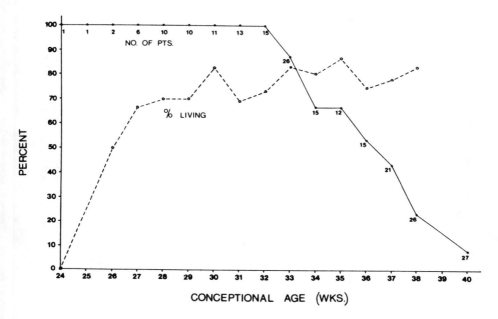

FIGURE 5.9 Incidence of quiescence in prematures. Note that all infants up to 32 weeks will show at least some quiescence and 50% of those at 36 weeks show the phenomenon. The dashed line shows the percent who remained alive at 3 years of age.

prematures (22 to 23 weeks), with an average duration of about 0.5 second, steadily declining to zero at term. Abnormality is indicated as a neurophysiological immaturity by the presence of many STOP patterns at term.

Premature temporal theta (PTθ)   The next distinctive pattern to emerge in the young premature is the PTθ pattern[24] (see Fig. 5.12). This pattern, like the STOP, is theta in frequency but often slightly slower at 4 to 5 c/sec, and also sharp in configuration, but one difference is that this pattern is nearly always (95%) bilateral in any given record and is clearly maximal on the *temporal* areas. This pattern can be seen in very young prematures but increases and peaks at 29 to 31 weeks and thereafter the incidence diminishes to zero at term. The duration is usually 1 to 1.5 seconds. As in STOP, abnormality is indicated as a neurophysiological immaturity by the presence of many examples of PTθ at term.

Sleep and Wake States

Active (rapid eye movement) sleep   In Figure 5.13, the reader is reminded that continuous activity may appear at approximately 32 weeks GA and

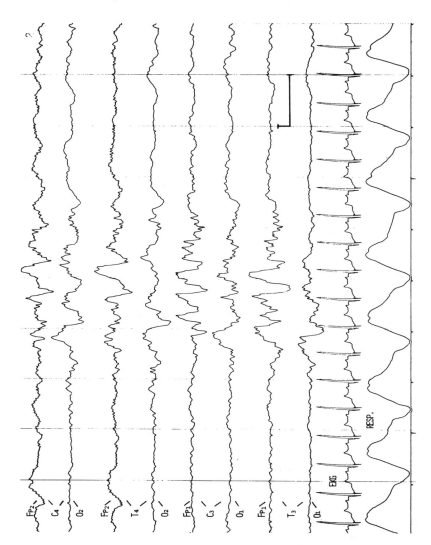

FIGURE 5.10 Tracé alternant pattern (NREM). This pattern (term baby, 1 week old) consists of bursts of activity interspersed between periods of decreased amplitude, but note that some activity can be seen during these latter periods.

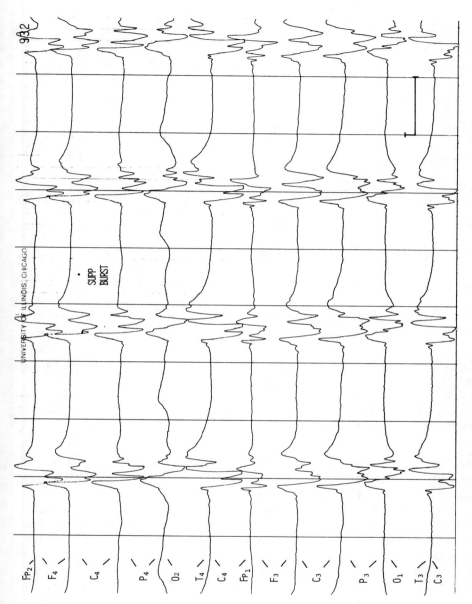

FIGURE 5.11 Suppression burst. This pattern consists of flat periods between periods of *high* amplitude activity from all regions, usually including *sharp* epileptiform deflections.

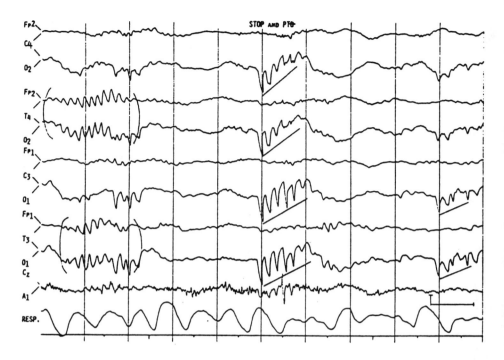

FIGURE 5.12   The STOP and PTθ patterns. Note the sharp theta bursts on Channels 2, 4, 6, and 8 (occipital areas) as an example of STOP and the theta bursts on Channels 3 and 4 (right temporal) and also 7 and 8 (left temporal) as an example of PTθ. (From Hughes JR, et al. Sharp theta rhythm on the occipital areas of premature. Clin EEG 1990; 21(2), with permission.)

after that time different stages of sleep begin to be organized. The first organized stage is active sleep (AS) or the rapid eye movement (REM) stage, appearing first at 32 weeks.[25] At this time and also throughout life, ONE OF THE CHARACTERISTIC FEATURES OF *AS* OR *REM* SLEEP IS THAT *CONTINUOUS* ACTIVITY APPEARS, CONSISTING MAINLY OF THE SAME FREQUENCIES AS APPEARED DISCONTINUOUSLY IN THE EARLIER AGES. Thus, very slow (0.3 to 1.0/sec) and very fast (8 to 30/sec) rhythms combine and are maximal usually on the occipital areas (Fig. 5.14). Another important identifying feature that now must be added is recorded by an electrode to monitor respiration, and also another electrode can be useful for monitoring the chin electromyogram (EMG). IN REM SLEEP *RESPIRATION* IS *IRREGULAR* AND THE *CHIN EMG* TRACING IS *QUIET*. Unlike the quiet chin EMG, however, the eyes are often moving.

Quiet (non-rapid eye movement) sleep   The quiet sleep (QS) or non–rapid eye movement (NREM) sleep first appears at approximately 34 weeks GA and becomes fully defined at 36 weeks[26] (see Fig. 5.13). In contradistinction to AS or REM sleep, with its continuous EEG activity, QS OR NREM NOW

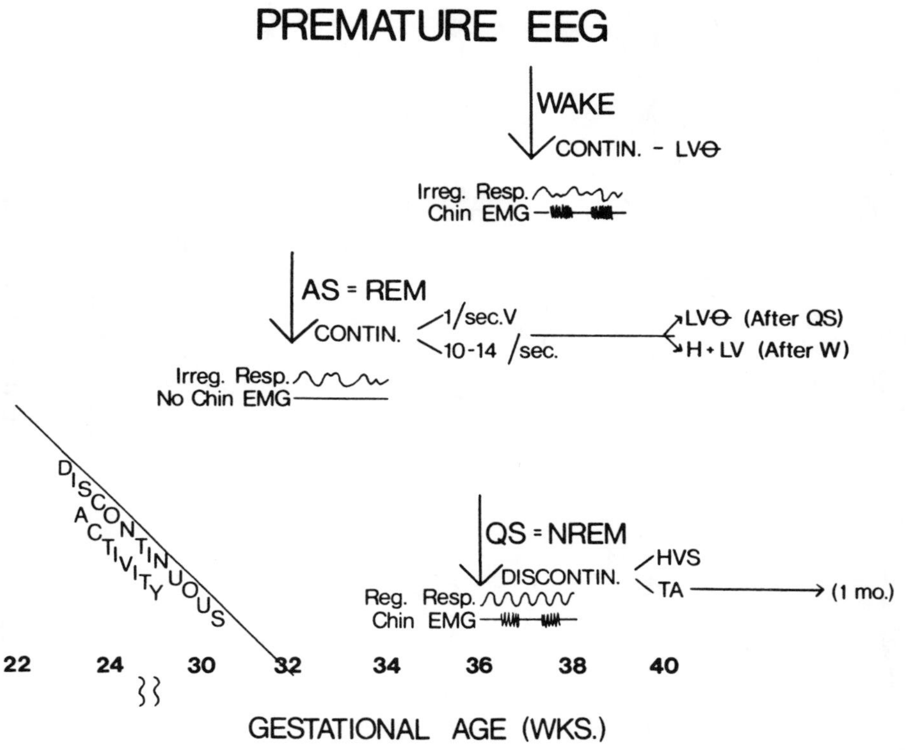

PREMATURE EEG

FIGURE 5.13 Summary of onset of different stages in the premature. Active sleep (AS) or rapid eye movement (REM) stage appears at 32 weeks with irregular respiration and quiet chin EMG. Around term this activity can be low voltage theta or mixed high and low voltage. Quiet sleep (QS) or non–rapid eye movement (NREM) stage begins at 34 weeks with regular respiration and chin EMG, seen either as high voltage slowing (HVS) or tracé alternant (TA), the latter remaining until 1 month past term. The waking (W) stage appears at 37 weeks with irregular respiration and chin EMG, characterized by low voltage theta (LVθ) rhythms.

SHOWS AND WILL SHOW THROUGHOUT LIFE *DISCONTINUOUS* FEATURES, mainly in the infant as the tracé alternant (TA), as seen in Figure 5.10. The second of the two patterns seen at this time is high voltage slow (HVS) activity at 1 to 2/sec (Fig. 5.15). The TA pattern will remain until the infant is approximately 1 month past term,[27] and the bursts of activity consist of many different components (1 to 3/sec waves, low voltage theta, and sharp transients), lasting up to 5 seconds in duration.

The physiological monitors will again be important in confirming QS or NREM sleep. AT THIS TIME AND THROUGHOUT LIFE RESPIRATION WILL BE REGULAR DURING NREM SLEEP; ALSO A *CHIN EMG* WILL USUALLY *APPEAR*, BUT NO EYE MOVEMENT WILL BE SEEN.

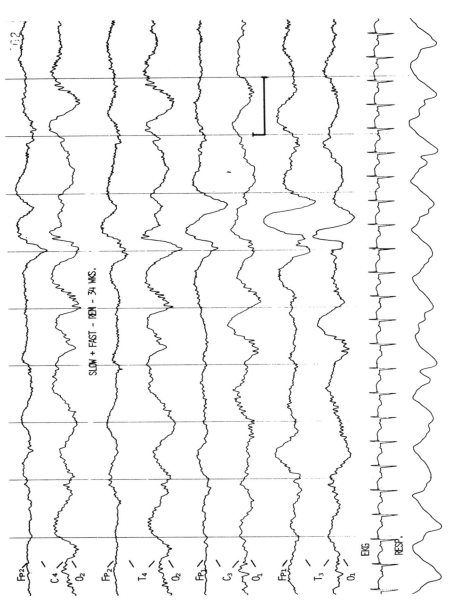

FIGURE 5.14   Very slow (0.5 to 1/sec) and very fast (10 to 25/sec) rhythms of REM or AS maximal on the occipital areas. GA = 34 weeks. Note irregularity of respiration (last channel).

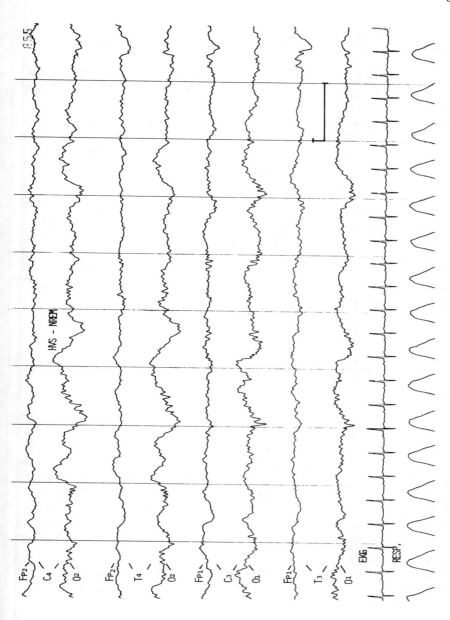

FIGURE 5.15 High voltage slow (HVS) in QS or NREM, consisting primarily of high voltage waves of 0.5 to 2/sec but fast, low amplitude activity can also be seen. Note very regular respiration (last channel). GA = 36 weeks.

Wake   At 37 weeks the waking (W) state will become organized,[28] consisting of low voltage theta (LVθ) activity, as seen in Figure 5.16, also called activité moyenne by the French.[29]

THE PHYSIOLOGICAL MONITORS DURING WAKE WILL SHOW *IRREGULAR RESPIRATION* AND (UNLIKE AS OR REM) A *CHIN EMG*, IN ADDITION TO OPEN EYES AND LIMB MOVEMENTS.

As a short summary, *regular* respiration will appear only in *QS or NREM. Irregular* respiration will appear either during *REM* or *wake*, but a *chin EMG* will differentiate the two by its absence during REM and presence during *wake. Continuous* EEG can be seen during *REM* or *wake* and *discontinuous* EEG may be seen during *NREM.*

Later activity   The REM stage is similar to the waking EEG at term and consists of LVθ (theta), especially when the REM appears after quiet sleep. If REM appears after wake a different pattern tends to be seen, namely, mixed high and low voltage (H + LV) rhythms (Fig. 5.17).[30]

At term, certain slow EEG patterns during wake can often be specified as clearly abnormal. These include continuous 1/sec rhythms and also long bursts of theta waves on a low voltage background.[31]

Symmetry

Not only among prematures, but for all ages, a consistent asymmetry greater than 2:1 in amplitude is abnormal on the side of the diminished amplitude.

Synchrony

When discontinuous activity occurs before 32 weeks, as seen in Fig. 5.7, the two hemispheres act somewhat independently and therefore asynchronous activity appears. Thus, the activity on one side of the head is completely different from that on the opposite side. Figure 5.18 shows that THE EARLIEST ACTIVITY AT *22 TO 23 WEEKS GA* IS ASSOCIATED WITH SYNCHRONY *LESS THAN ONE-HALF OF THE TIME* AND WITH INCREASING AGE, MORE SYNCHRONY APPEARS SO THAT AT TERM NEARLY 100% OF THE TIME SYNCHRONIZED RHYTHMS WILL APPEAR BETWEEN THE TWO SIDES OF THE HEAD (see Fig. 5.18).[32] Abnormality would be indicated by many examples (>25%) of asynchrony of the *major* rhythms at term.

Delta Brushes (DB)

The term *delta brush* refers to the combination of very slow *delta* waves plus fast activity, looking like hairs on a *brush* (see Fig. 5.19). As Figure 5.20 shows, immature (abortive) DELTA BRUSHES APPEAR AS EARLY AS 28 WEEKS GA, BECOME PROMINENT AT 32 WEEKS, and are USUALLY

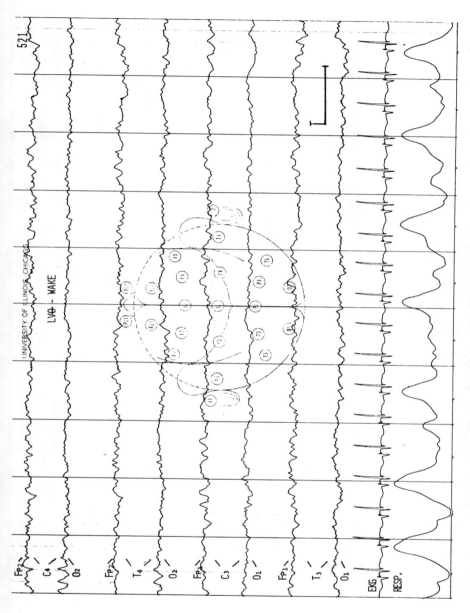

FIGURE 5.16 Waking record with low voltage theta (LVθ). Term infant, 3 days old. Note irregularity of respiration (last channel). Some slower rhythms and alpha components can also be noted.

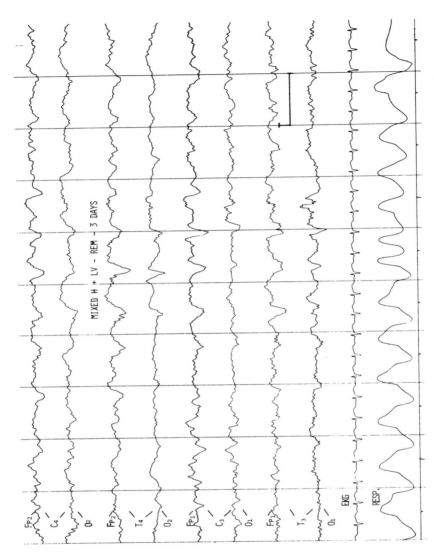

FIGURE 5.17   Mixed high and low voltage (H + LV) pattern characteristic of REM (term). Age = term + 3 days. Note high voltage slow waves (delta) and also low voltage activity (theta). Also, irregular respiration can be seen on the last channel.

PREMATURE EEG

DEGREE (%) OF SYNCHRONY

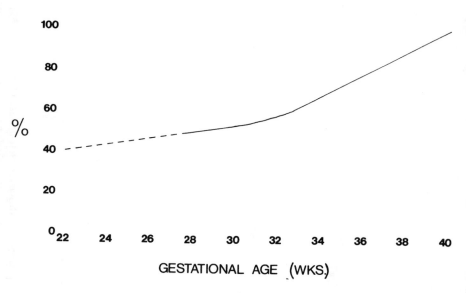

FIGURE 5.18 Synchrony between two hemispheres in the premature. The line shows an increasing synchrony from 22 to 23 weeks GA until near term. The dashed portion indicates that the data are somewhat scanty.

GONE AT TERM.[33] If DB are found more often than 2 every 10 seconds at term, they should be considered excessive and therefore abnormal.

Sharp Activity

Sporadic sharp waves The most difficult aspect of interpreting premature EEGs is likely the evaluation of sharp activity. If an adult shows a clear spike discharge on a given area, this activity can usually be considered abnormal and reported as such. In the premature, the simple presence or absence of such spikes or sharp waves usually does not designate the pattern as abnormal but instead IT IS MORE THE *EXTENT* OF SUCH ACTIVITY THAT DETERMINES ABNORMALITY. The reason that this difficult judgment must be made is that some sharp waves, called *sporadic sharp waves,* do normally occur in premature infants (see Fig. 5.21).[34] THESE SHARP WAVES DO APPEAR SPORADICALLY (HERE AND THERE, NOW AND THEN ON DIFFERENT AREAS), FIRST MAKING THEIR APPEARANCE AT 30 WEEKS (see Fig. 5.22), BECOMING PROMINENT ESPECIALLY ON THE CENTRAL AREAS AT 40 WEEKS, AND OFTEN APPEARING IN QS

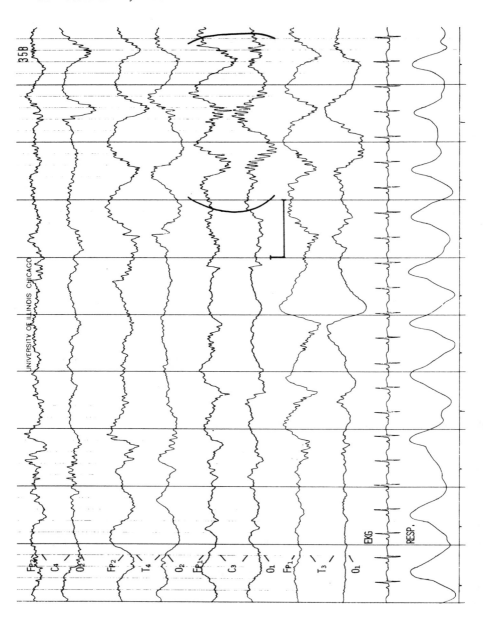

FIGURE 5.19   Delta brushes (DB). These patterns (outlined) consist of sharp fast activity superimposed on slow delta waves. GA = 32 weeks.

PREMATURE EEG

DELTA BRUSHES

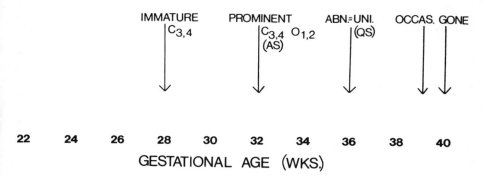

FIGURE 5.20   Changes in delta brushes with age.

AT 1 WEEK PAST TERM AND THEN USUALLY GONE AT 8 WEEKS OR 2 MONTHS. Thus, each of the (negative) sharp waves after 2 months of age can be treated as other sharp waves in the child and adult and designated as abnormal, regardless of how frequently they appear.

Abnormal sharp waves   The abnormal sharp wave (negative) as seen in Figure 5.22, differs from the normal sporadic variety by its persistence (see Fig. 5.23) since IT CONSISTENTLY AND REPEATEDLY APPEARS ON A GIVEN FOCAL REGION AS EARLY AS 30 WEEKS GA. The number required to qualify as abnormal from a given region is between 1/min[35] and 2/min[36] from that same region. One particular variety of sharp wave that is blunted in its appearance and often repetitive is called a *burnt-out sharp wave*[37] (Fig. 5.24); these discharges can be considered abnormal.

Frontal sharp transients   Another form of sharp activity that is characteristic of the premature EEG is the frontal sharp transient,[38] as seen in Figure 5.25. As noted in Fig. 5.22, THIS PATTERN (CALLED *ENCOCHES FRONTALES* BY THE FRENCH) MAY APPEAR VERY EARLY AT 26 WEEKS, IS PROMINENT WITH ANTERIOR DELTA RHYTHMS AT 36 WEEKS, AND LIKELY REMAINS IN SLEEP STATES FOR 1 MONTH PAST TERM. The appearance of these transients, often seen in transition between active and quiet sleep, predicts a favorable outcome. However, when they are abundant, long in duration, and high in amplitude, they may represent minor pathology, especially from stressed babies.[39]

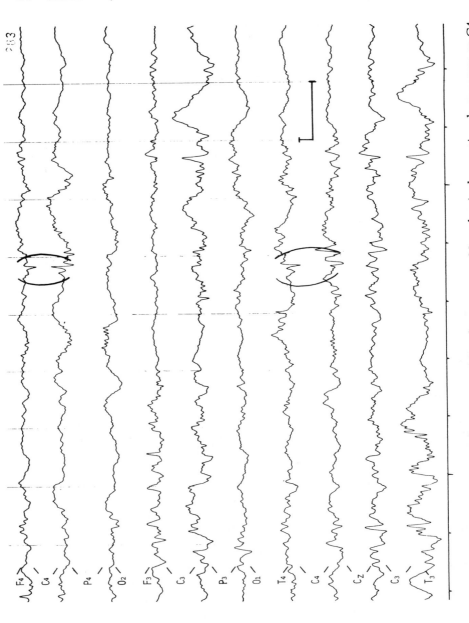

FIGURE 5.21   Sporadic sharp waves, normal in the premature. Note the single negative sharp waves on C4 electrode, which rarely appeared. Term + 2 weeks.

PREMATURE & POST-NATAL EEG

SHARP ACTIVITY

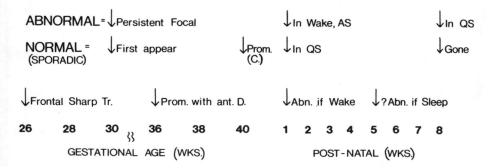

FIGURE 5.22 Summary of sharp waves with age, including the (normal) sporadic sharp waves, the (abnormal) persistent sharp waves, and frontal sharp transients (Fr. sh. tr.).

A useful summary of the premature EEG appears in Figure 5.26, showing the normal limits for the most prominent types of activity seen at the different conceptional ages.

THE SIMPLEST SUMMARY OF THE PREMATURE EEG IS THAT THE EARLIEST ACTIVITY IS THE COMBINATION OF FAST AND SLOW RHYTHMS, DISCONTINUOUS UNTIL 32 WEEKS, OFTEN CONTINUOUS AFTER THAT TIME. THE EARLIEST DISTINCTIVE PATTERN IS THE STOP (WITH QUIESCENCE), FOLLOWED BY THE PTθ PATTERN WITH MAXIMAL REPRESENTATION AT 29 TO 31 WEEKS. AT 36 WEEKS GA, WAKE AND ACTIVE SLEEP SHOWS LOW VOLTAGE THETA (LVθ) AND QUIET SLEEP SHOWS TRACÉ ALTERNANT (TA) AND HIGH VOLTAGE SLOW (HVS). AT TERM, DELTA BRUSHES (DB) ARE GONE, AT 1 MONTH FRONTAL SHARP TRANSIENTS AND TA DISAPPEAR, AND AT 2 MONTHS SPORADIC SHARP WAVES ARE ABSENT.

Other related changes Some other related points can be added to this discussion of the premature period. Some authors have claimed that the short period of time between 28 and 29 weeks GA is a time when theta rhythms synchronized within one hemisphere can appear.[40] Some investigators have attempted to determine the physiological parameter that is the most reliable measure of the state of the premature. Although a matter of opinion, some authors have maintained that reliability comes best from body movement at 28 weeks, eye movement at 32 weeks, the EEG itself at 36 weeks,

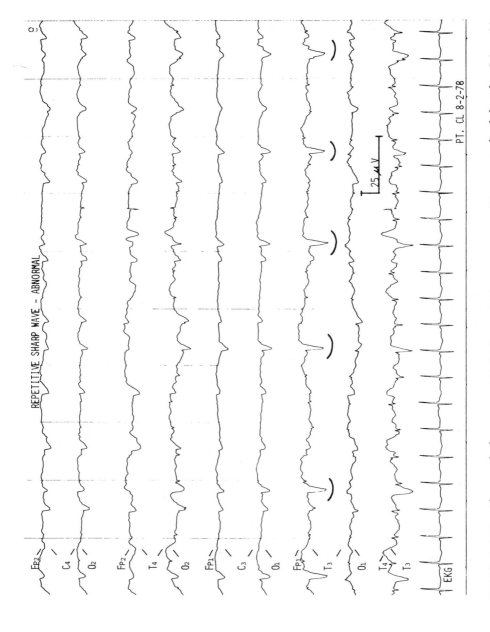

FIGURE 5.23   Abnormal sharp wave. Note its repetitiveness or persistence on the left side. GA = 38 weeks.

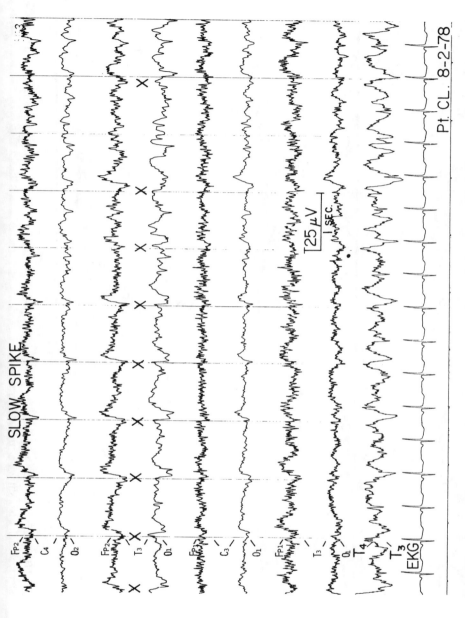

FIGURE 5.24 Burnt-out sharp wave. Note the dulled or blunted negative phase, which is also prolonged or slow. GA = 38 weeks.

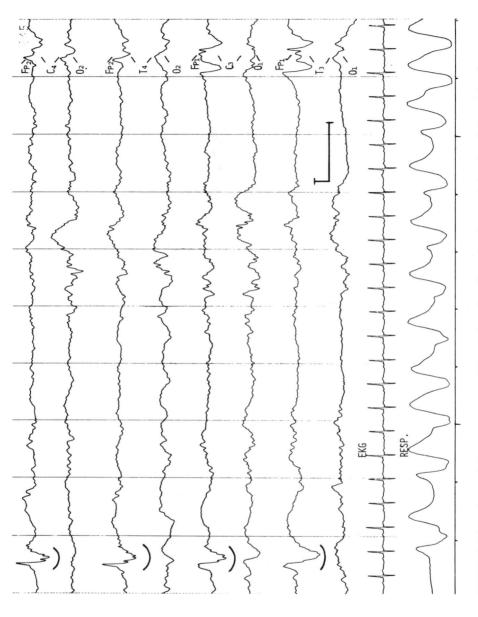

FIGURE 5.25 Frontal sharp transient. GA = 36 weeks. Note the slow activity that follows the sharp transient, which also shows a minor asymmetry.

SUMMARY OF PREMATURES & NEONATES

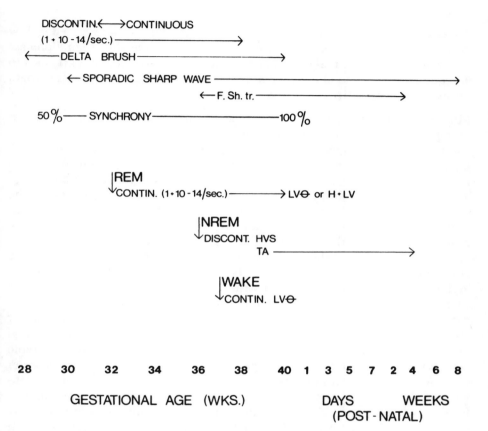

FIGURE 5.26   Summary of the premature and the characteristic activity appearing at different ages. See text for details.

and chin movement at 40 weeks.[41] Since spontaneous EEG activity is intrinsically related to evoked potentials (EP), a few words on EP are in order. As early as 28 weeks CA a monophasic visual EP can appear, which becomes triphasic at 32 weeks.[42] From auditory stimulation a vertex negative sharp deflection can appear as early as 30 weeks[43] and peaks I and V of the brain stem auditory evoked potential can usually be seen at that time.

EEG of Neonates, Young Infants, and Children (to Adult)

As the premature infant becomes older beyond term into the neonatal stage, EEG changes continue to appear, but not so rapidly as during the premature period. This section deals with the characteristic patterns during this neo-natal period of development and how they change with age up to childhood.

Wake

Theta and alpha.   The waking record at birth (term) is characterized by low voltage theta rhythms, especially on the central regions, but then alpha activity at 8 to 13 c/sec makes its appearance posteriorly, often as early as 3 to 4 years.[3] In time, the alpha increases in prominence and the central theta diminishes so that little remains by adolescence.

Mu   This pattern usually does not appear in infants but has been described in approximately 7% of healthy children.[44] Mu has been called "en arceau" rhythm because its appearance is arclike. These waves come in bursts, lasting from a few up to many seconds, and are maximal on the central (C3, C4) regions, often appearing on one side at a time but usually seen on both sides at some time throughout the record. They have a sharp negativity on the central regions and bipolar recordings incorporating the C3, C4 areas can reveal sharp phase reversals that can easily leave a mistaken impression of a burst of rhythmical epileptiform activity. Their frequency is within the alpha range, but often they are slightly (within 1/sec) faster than the more sinusoidal alpha appearing posteriorly.[45] In contradistinction to posterior alpha responsive mainly to visual stimuli, mu waves are mainly responsive to movements or thought of movements of the opposite extremity, but they can disappear or desynchronize with many other kinds of maneuvers or stimulations (Fig. 5.27). Although considered by most electroencephalographers as a normal pattern, they may represent a relatively hyperexcitable state within the central regions, especially since they can be the forerunner of some focal discharges that can later appear from the same region.[46] A single mu wave can be so sharp that its differentiation from a focal epileptiform spike from the C3 and C4 area can be most difficult, but the best judgment at this time is to deal with mu waves conservatively and call them normal. Some electroencephalographers have maintained that their *absence* on one side is evidence for an abnormality on that same side in the same way that a significant depression of (normal) alpha would argue for an abnormality on that side,[47] but more recent evidence indicates that their *presence* on only one side indicates pathology on that same side.[48]

Sleep

In REM sleep a low voltage *theta* gives way more to a low voltage *fast* pattern at 3 months, and this pattern will continue throughout life.[49] In NREM, drowsiness in the young infant is often seen as increasing amplitudes with decreasing frequencies down to 2 to 3 c/sec maximal on the occipital areas.[17] At 3 years, frontal theta waves appear during drowsiness, remaining throughout adulthood.[17] Finally, fast rhythms at 20 to 28 c/sec

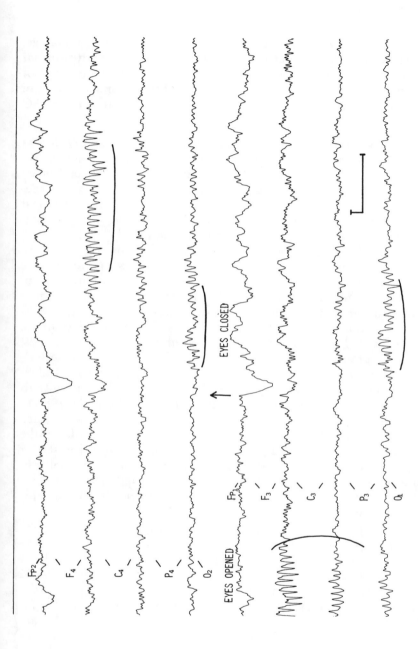

FIGURE 5.27 Mu waves. These waves are similar in frequency to the alpha, but are maximal on the central (C$_{3,4}$) areas, responding especially to movements of the contralateral limb. Note that the mu waves, seen on Channels 2 and 3 on the right side and 6 and 7 on the left side, appear during eyes open when the alpha on Channels 4 and 8 has disappeared. The alpha then reappears only after the closing of the eyes. The mu and alpha are therefore independent rhythms.

become prominent at 1 year and are usually present until 5–6 years of age, when they disappear.[3] This fast activity should not be confused with similar frequencies that are seen in patients taking medication of the barbiturate or benzodiazepine type, nor should their presence in children under 6 years of age be attributed to chloral hydrate, often given as a sleep aid in the EEG laboratory.

Spindles   Spindles are characteristic of stage II sleep and usually appear throughout the lifetime of all normal individuals. As Figure 5.28 shows, rudimentary spindles with some 14/sec activity can appear as early as 1 week past term but clear 14/sec spindles are first seen at 1.5 to 2 months especially at 6 weeks. At 3 months, an interesting change occurs which may last only a few months. These spindles are very long in duration, at times lasting more than 10 seconds, and are biphasic in appearance.[17]

At 5 months of age, the spindles are shorter in duration but asynchronous, appearing only on one side at a time.[17] Another change is that they are monophasic in appearance, meaning that they have an accentuated sharpness in the negative phase. On a monopolar or referential montage, these spindles (from frontal-central areas) show a sharpness in the upward direction. On a bipolar montage along parasagittal areas, as seen in the example of Figure 5.29, they show a phase reversal around the C3, C4 electrodes, again reflecting a prominent negativity on those electrodes. Characteristically, they show a near-equipotentiality on the central and parietal electrodes, so that their appearance may be nearly absent on this linkage with only a small deflection on the parietal–occipital linkage (see Fig. 5.29). On such a bipolar, parasagittal montage the characteristic appearance is sharp downward deflections at 14/sec on the frontal-central linkage looking like 14/sec positive spikes, *if* that linkage had been referential from the posterior temporal area to the contralateral ear. One can find published examples in the literature of events that were called 14/sec positive spikes in young infants, which in reality are normal asynchronous monophasic 14/sec spindles from a frontal-central linkage.[50]

At 1 year, as seen in Figure 5.28, asynchronous spindles should disappear as the commissural pathways linking both halves of the brain become more mature and active. At 1 year of age, the *majority* of spindles should be synchronous between the two sides and, at 2 years of age, nearly *all* should be synchronous; otherwise, they likely represent an abnormality within the thalamocortical projection system. The usual biphasic appearance of spindles that remains for the rest of life is seen around the age of 3 years.[51] Only one other change normally occurs with spindles and this change is the addition of 12/sec spindles at age 5 years, remaining into the teens, in addition to the 14/sec form.[3]

K-complex   The term K-complex refers to the combination of the normal vertex slow or sharp transient and the spindle, appearing apparently spontaneously or in response to a sudden stimulus. As seen in Figure 5.30, this

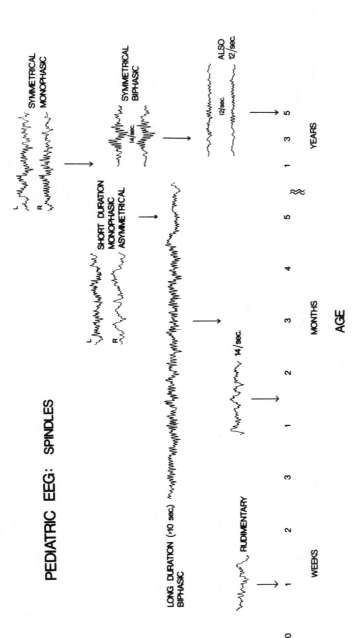

FIGURE 5.28   Spindles and their change in the infant. First, rudimentary activity is seen; later, long-lasting and biphasic; then asymmetrical and monophasic; later, symmetrical; and, still later, biphasic spindles of the adult form appear.

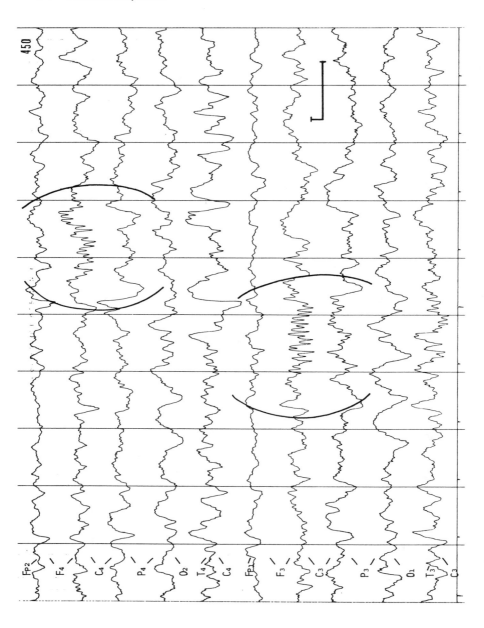

FIGURE 5.29   Asymmetrical monophasic spindles on a bipolar montage. Note the frontocentral linkage with its characteristic downward sharpness. Age = 8 months.

PEDIATRIC EEG

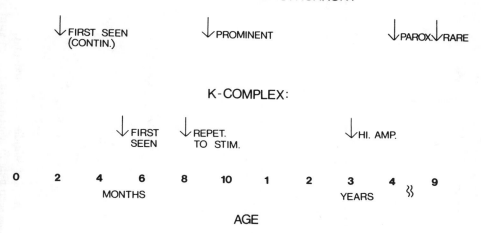

FIGURE 5.30   Changes in hypnagogic hypersynchrony and K-complexes with age. See text for details.

electrographic pattern appears first at 5 months, but then at 8 months the sharp transient portion of the K-complex may appear repetitively in response to a given stimulus[52] (see Fig. 5.31). The amplitude of this pattern increases in age, so that at age 3 years,[3] high amplitudes appear, remaining high for the next 5 years but also appearing prominent until the early teens.

Hypnagogic hypersynchrony   The term *hypnagogic hypersynchrony* refers to very synchronous activity appearing usually in early drowsiness but also at times during arousal from deeper sleep.[53] As noted in Figure 5.30, this phenomenon first appears at the age of 2 months and at that time consists of high amplitude, continuous delta rhythms (or θ)[54] (Fig. 5.32). These latter rhythms become prominent at 9 months,[55] but at age 4 years they become shorter in duration and more paroxysmal in appearance[56] (Fig. 5.33). At age 9 years hypnagogic hypersynchrony becomes rare.

Summary   Figure 5.34 provides a summary of the EEG of the neonate, infant, and child. The waking record at birth is characterized by low voltage theta rhythms, but then later alpha activity makes its appearance over the occipital areas. In REM, the low voltage fast pattern appearing at 3 months will continue throughout life. In NREM, drowsiness is often seen as increasing amplitudes of delta waves, and, at 3 years of age, frontal theta appears during drowsiness, remaining throughout adulthood.

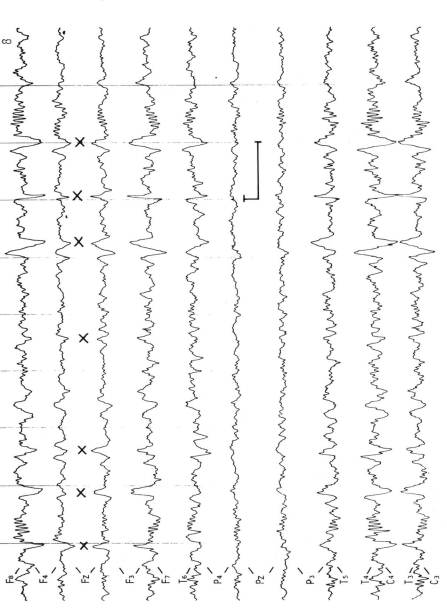

FIGURE 5.31 K-complex. The vertex sharp transient plus spindles, as noted in text, constitute a K-complex. The sharp component can be repetitive, as seen here in response to a given stimulus.

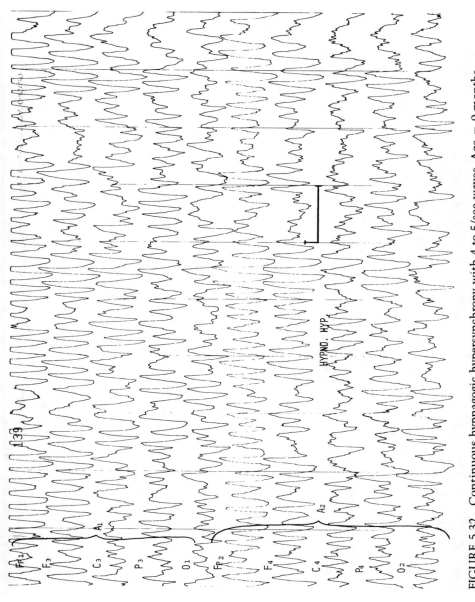

FIGURE 5.32 Continuous hypnagogic hypersynchrony with 4 to 5/sec waves. Age = 9 months.

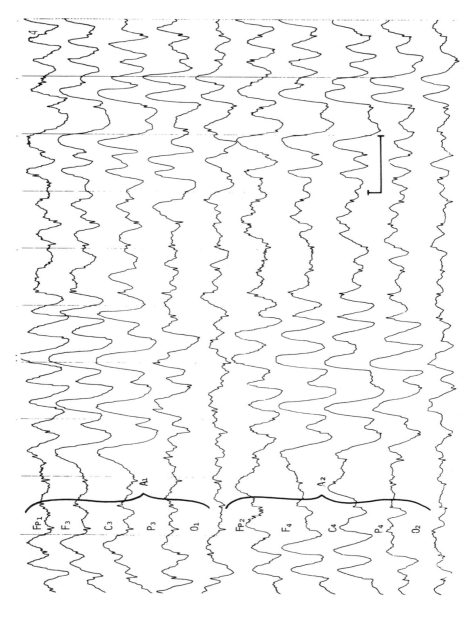

FIGURE 5.33   Paroxysmal hypnagogic hypersynchrony. Note the bursts of high amplitude delta waves during drowsiness. Age = 4 years.

SUMMARY OF INFANTS & CHILDREN

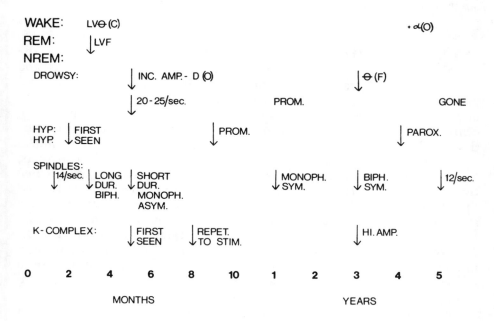

FIGURE 5.34 Summary of the EEG of the neonate, infant and child. See text for details.

Elderly

Wake

The EEG of the waking elderly patient is similar to that of the adult, except that the frequency of the alpha rhythm tends to decrease with age.[6] The average frequency of the background rhythm in healthy centenarians, however, is still over 8 c/sec[7] and, therefore, slower frequencies in the elderly can be considered abnormal, mild in degree if 7 to 7.5 c/sec, moderate if under 7 but over 6 s/sec, and marked if under 6 c/sec.

Sleep

The sleep rhythms in healthy elderly individuals are essentially similar to those in adults, except that very rapid changes in the state of awareness are noted in these senior citizens. Alpha activity, representing wakefulness, can appear within seconds of sleep spindles, representing stage II sleep, as an example of quick shifts of stages of alertness.

Summary—All Ages

Figure 5.35 shows a summary of all of the major normal patterns from infancy to 16 yrs of age, the latter similar to the adult in EEG development.

Wake

This figure shows the mean frequency of the background rhythm on the *occipital* areas increasing from 5 to 6 c/sec (1 yr) to 7 to 8 c/sec (2 yrs) and 9 c/sec (9 yrs) to 10 c/sec (15 yrs). Abnormally slow background rhythms are usually those that are 1.5 c/sec slower than the mean for infants and children and those under 8 c/sec for everyone at least 8 years of age. The *fronto-central* theta rhythms are often 6 to 7 c/sec, slightly higher in frequency than the 5 to 6 c/sec waves on the occipital areas of the 1-year-old infant. An increasing incidence is seen at 6 years, the highest amplitude at 8 years, bursts at 9 years, with the highest incidence at 13 to 14 years, after which they decrease. Abnormality is indicated by high amplitude theta ($>$100 µV) that dominates over the posterior alpha or the presence of any clear theta after the mid-20s. *Mu* waves are rare in children with a peak in early adolescence and are seen more often in females but noted in only about 20%. Abnormality is indicated by strictly unilateral mu. *Beta* rhythms are seen in one-quarter of pre-teens, are usually low in amplitude, and increase in incidence in mid-teens. Abnormality is indicated if these waves are completely depressed on one side. *Posterior slow waves* are rare at 1 year, develop as slow transients in the next few years, are maximal in the female at 5 years and in the male at 9 years, then decrease to 15% in the mid-teens and are gone by the early 20s. Abnormality is indicated by the presence of bursts of rhythmical delta waves, as opposed to polyphasic slow transients. Normal posterior slow waves can also appear in two other forms. One is "alpha variant," referring to subharmonics of alpha ($\frac{1}{2}$ the frequency) so that 10 c/sec waves are seen intermixed with 5 c/sec rhythms, seen as early as preteens. Also, a specific (uncommon) slow rhythm at 2.5 to 4.5 c/sec can appear[44] especially at 5 to 7 years of age, and be gone at 15 years. The difference between this pattern and the abnormal bursts is that the normal type is low in amplitude ($<$100 µV) in short bursts ($<$3 sec) and is nonfocal over the entire posterior scalp region, while the abnormal type is usually high in amplitude, in long bursts maximal on the occipital areas. *Lambda* waves are similar to visual evoked potentials in that they are seen on the occipital areas, usually with both negative and positive phases, in response to eye movements, especially when the stimulus is "interesting." They can often be seen best in children 2 to 3 years of age, possibly because of a thinner skull than in adults, and slowly decrease in preteens and teens. Abnormality is indicated by a depression on one side. *Photic* driving can be seen at frequencies $<$8/sec around 8 to 9 years and then up to 15 to 20/sec after 10 to 11 years of age.

Hyperventilation changes (Fig. 5.3) that are diffuse are maximal on the occipital areas in younger children (5 to 6 years) and on the frontal areas in

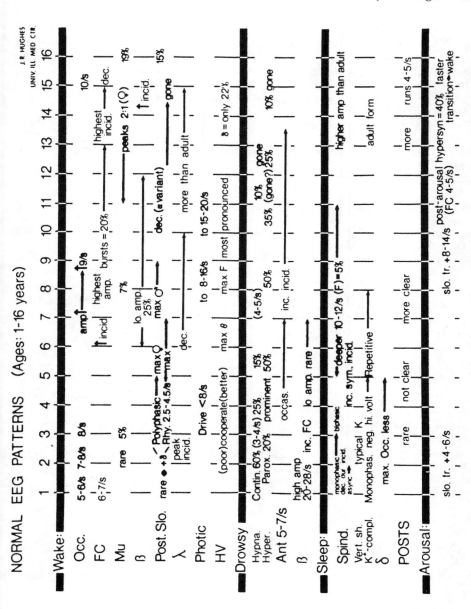

FIGURE 5.35 Summary of normal patterns in wake, drowsy, sleep, and arousal. See text for details.

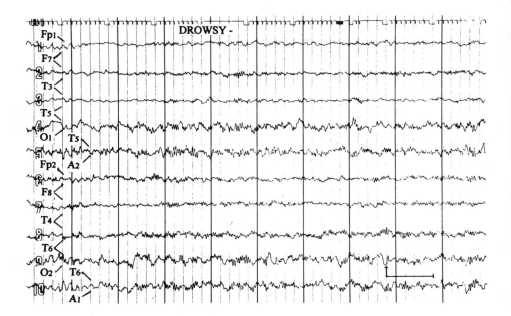

FIGURE 5.36 Fast activity during drowsiness in infants and young children. Note the 22 to 28/sec activity, appearing diffusely, but best seen posteriorly (Channels 4 and 5, 9 and 10). Patient is 3 years old.

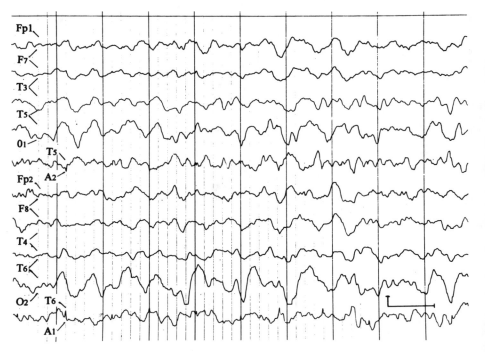

FIGURE 5.37 Cone-shaped delta waves on the occipital areas during sleep in young children. Note on Channels 4 (left) and 9 (right) the high amplitude slow waves that, at times, are cone-shaped.

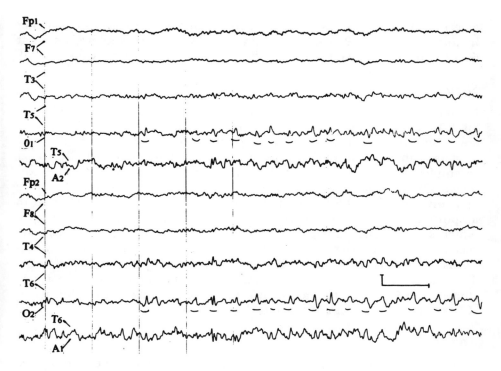

FIGURE 5.38 Positive occipital sharp transients of sleep (POSTS). Note on Channels 4 (left) and 9 (right) the sharp upward deflections (underlined) that may appear as a single event or in bursts. The linkage of posterior temporal to occipital with an upward sharp deflection means that the occipital areas were relatively positive (negative to positive = up).

older preteens. Abnormality is indicated only by focal findings or diffuse epileptiform patterns.

Drowsy

Figure 5.35 also shows the normal drowsy patterns. *Hypnagogic hypersynchrony* comes in two forms, the earliest as a continuous form (Fig. 5.32) at 3 to 4 c/sec and maximal at 2 years on the posterior regions. They decrease in incidence thereafter, increasing in frequency to 4 to 5 c/sec at 7 to 8 years on the frontal areas. The paroxysmal form (Fig. 5.33) starts later at around 3 years, is prominent at 5 to 9 years, and decreases thereafter. Both of these forms are gone in the early teens; the paroxysmal form starts slightly later and lasts slightly longer. Abnormality is indicated by these forms appearing in the late teens. *Anterior* theta waves at 5 to 7 c/sec are occasionally seen in young children, increasing in incidence with older age. This anterior rhythm in drowsiness can also be seen at times in the alpha or even beta range, and rarely as delta waves; the latter is occasionally noted in the elderly.[57] As the last drowsy pattern *beta* rhythm at 20 to 28 c/sec is higher in amplitude at 1 to 2 years of age, lower at 4 to 5 years, and rarely seen at 6 to 7 years. They are often maximal on the posterior regions (see Fig. 5.36).

Sleep

In Figure 5.35 sleep rhythms are also noted. *Spindles* (Fig. 5.28) at 14 c/sec are at first monophasic and asynchronous, becoming synchronous at 2 years and biphasic at 3 years. In deeper sleep they may be seen at 10 to 12 c/sec, especially in children; in the preteens and teens spindles are usually higher in amplitude than in the adult. *Vertex sharp transients and K-complexes* (Fig. 5.31) can be seen in the young infant, becoming typical at 2 to 3 years and very repetitive at 5 to 8 years of age. The adult form, which is lower in amplitude and is nonrepetitive, is seen in the early teens. *Delta* waves, which are cone-shaped (Fig. 5.37) and maximal on the occipital areas, are seen at 2 years but disappear at 5 to 6 years. One of the most evident waveforms in sleep is the *POST*[58] (positive occipital sharp transients of sleep). This pattern is rare at 3 years, is clearer at 8 years, and begins to appear in runs at 4 to 5 c/sec in the mid-teens; it develops further in the adult when it is a dominant rhythm in Stage II sleep (Fig. 5.38).

Arousal

In infants an arousal is often followed by slow transients and 4 to 6 c/sec waves. Later at 8 to 10 yrs these frequencies often are higher at 8 to 14 c/sec. The frequencies that typify arousal from sleep into wakefulness can generally be called "postarousal hypersynchrony." The frontocentral location of 4 to 5 c/sec rhythms is often seen in adolescents (40%)[50] and young adults.

CHAPTER 6

Abnormal Rhythms

General Comments

A colleague of mine once sang the praises of an old-time electroencephalographer by stating that a designation of an abnormal EEG by that electroencephalographer essentially meant a brain tumor. Instead of an accolade, this comment may have really been an indictment that many subtle patterns were missed and mistakenly called normal. The major point here is that EEG abnormality varies in degree as much as anything else varies—from very mild to very severe. Electroencephalographers draw different lines as to the point at which a pattern or finding is called abnormal, but most agree that the "borderline EEG" offers no help to the clinician and should be avoided. Another way to make the major point here is to state that the electroencephalographer should grade the abnormality in some way that is understandable to the clinician, in the hope of avoiding terms such as grade I, II, and III, requiring a ready reference to remind one which is the worst, I or III. Progress in all fields can often be defined by the discovery of subtleties, rather than an appreciation of only the grossest, most obvious findings, and EEG is no exception. Electroencephalographers, however, are often reluctant to label some of these "subtleties" as abnormal, because so many clinicians still believe any "abnormal EEG" is ominous and often tantamount to a diagnosis of epilepsy. Education of the electroencephalographers to recognize some of these patterns and of the clinicians to appreciate their significance, at times only minor, but often adding helpful information, is a problem of the future.

The EEG should be viewed as a test that provides evidence for or against an organic or physical brain abnormality. At times, this evidence is weak and at other times strong. The report of the electroencephalographer can be phrased to take into account this variable of degree, and the clinician should be made somewhat aware of the extent of evidence in favor of an abnormality. Since EEG can be considered as a test providing *evidence* for or against an organic brain abnormality, the same kind of terminology is useful in describing a "normal" EEG. Thus, the summary impression of a record without any abnormal features can be stated as showing *no evidence* for any abnormality, rather than using the phrase "normal EEG." This latter phrase too often may lead the clinician to conclude that the entire brain *must* therefore be normal physiologically and pathologically; also, the phrase "normal EEG" can lead to complex legal discussions in the courtroom.

Depression of Normal Rhythms

Cautions

Technical problems that interfere with the accurate recording of the true brain waves should always be under consideration by the electroencephalographer in the determination of any abnormality, but in assessing one particular form of abnormality, viz., the depression of normal rhythms, this consideration has special importance. Except in the records from laboratories with skilled technicians who routinely measure electrode resistance and require low values, "depressed" activity may be an artifact from an electrode of high resistance, which can reduce the amplitude of the rhythms it records. Correct identification of this latter kind of artifact can be difficult for the electroencephalographer who reads tracings from technicians who record with high resistance electrodes of varying values. A clue, however, that a depression is likely artificial is that the low amplitude is seen from only one electrode (with high resistance); a genuine depression of brain rhythms usually appears on more than one electrode, since most EEG abnormalities of *any* type usually spread beyond one single electrode. The electroencephalographer must also be certain that calibration was properly done and that the depression of rhythms in given channels cannot be from unequal gain or amplification in those same channels. One way to avoid a misinterpretation that a decreased amplitude represents abnormality rather than an improper gain that has developed on one or more channels is to use a sequence of montages that alternate the left and right sides on the top and bottom channels. Thus, if the top two channels recording from the left side suddenly show a decreased amplitude in the middle of the record and the next montage places the right side on the top channels which continue to show the depression on those same channels, the "depression" is a technical problem of those channels. If the depression remains on the left and moves with the montage, then the decreased amplitude is not a channel problem, but is either a faulty electrode or is a genuine depression of activity.

Other cautions must be mentioned. One point is that abnormal EEGs are rarely seen in the form of *only* a depression of normal activity; therefore, as the *only* finding in a record, such a decreased amplitude may be suspect. Also, a genuine depression should be consistent throughout the entire tracing, appearing similarly on all montages. This type of check will avoid the trap of mislabeling a decreased amplitude of activity as a depression of activity, when, in fact, it may be only a near-equipotentiality between two electrodes recording similar voltages and linked together in a bipolar manner to record their differences. Throughout a series of montages, a given electrode should be linked with different electrodes in both the anterior-posterior and the coronal directions and then equipotentialities will not likely continue to appear, since they rarely are seen between more than two given electrodes. Thus, the "depression" on one side will disappear with a new montage and can then be properly appreciated as an equipotentiality.

One last caution is that a genuine decrease in amplitude of background activity is often seen on the (left) dominant hemisphere, especially of right-handers, and a 50% difference in the peak to peak amplitude of the two sides is likely required before a consideration of abnormality is entertained from the side with the decreased rhythms. As was previously stated, depressions on the right are usually more significant and then a consistent 50% decrease in amplitude on the (nondominant) right side, especially of right-handers, may be considered as significant.

Collections of Fluid under Electrodes

A decreased amplitude of activity can be expected when the recording electrode is moved away from the source of that activity. Collections of fluid (blood, lymph, CSF, or any type) that separate the recording electrode from the brain can be expected to (and do) result in a decrease in amplitude of activity. Thus, subgaleal collections of fluid under the outer scalp but over the skull can result in a depression, as can epidural or subdural hematomas or hygromas. In the latter instance of subdural hematoma, the elegant term *hypopotentia* refers to this decreased amplitude, which likely occurs early in the chronology of events associated with subdurals, possibly before definite clinical signs appear. When the pressure from this fluid collection reaches a certain point, however, then clinical signs appear and the patient may be referred for an EEG. By that time, the increasing pressure has likely caused a significant neurophysiological disturbance of those neurones underlying the collection and slow wave abnormalities *also* usually appear. Thus, although a decreased amplitude of activity is often expected in patients with subdural collections, slow waves are the most common finding since depression of activity as the *only* positive EEG finding is somewhat uncommon in these patients.[59]

Other Conditions

In the same way that a depression of activity may be an early sign of abnormality in the case of subdural (or epidural) collections of fluid, such a depression may be an early sign of *any kind of abnormal condition*. For example, tumors may appear early in the EEG, only as a focal depression of activity[60] before revealing themselves by more impressive EEG findings, such as high amplitude slow waves. Furthermore, when tumors have reached this latter stage, they usually also show a depression of background activity, in addition to the slowing. European authors[61] have more often stressed the importance of this depression of activity than American investigators, and such an emphasis is likely a correct one. Similarly, a CVA often reveals itself both by slow waves and a depression of activity on the same side, but some authors believe that the combination of these two kinds of findings is related to a poorer prognosis than just the presence of slow waves alone.[62] Thus, a significantly decreased amplitude of activity, either focal or diffusely unilateral, rarely occurs by itself and should be considered a nonspecific finding. When such a finding appears in conjunction with other abnormalities, such as slow waves, the depression only confirms further the presence of abnormality and likely adds to the severity of the pathological condition.

The unilateral depression of 14 c/sec sleep spindles in stage II sleep can be considered as reflecting a disturbance in the thalamocortical pathways from the anterior diencephalon to the frontal cortex. At times, the pathology may lie at the level of the diencephalon and show up on the EEG only as a unilateral depression of frontocentral spindle activity without affecting the more posteriorly located alpha rhythms. Theoretically, an asymmetry of spindles can reflect pathology anywhere between the diencephalon and cortex, but often this finding appears with subcortical disorders.[63]

The unilateral depression of another form of "fast" activity can be used as a sign of abnormality. This fast activity is the beta rhythm that may occur frontally, especially in tense patients, but also rhythms at 20 to 25 c/sec related to barbiturate or benzodiazepine medication. Since this fast activity can be considered "normal," its depression can be considered abnormal. Years ago, confirmation of the side involved in a temporal lobe epilepsy was determined by injecting a barbiturate and checking which temporal area showed a depression of beta.[64] This test is now considered as nonspecific, but it does underscore the point that depression of normal activity is one form of an EEG abnormality.

When the two sides, left and right, are compared for amplitude differences of normal rhythms, the lower amplitude may not always reflect the abnormal side. In the instance of a previous craniotomy, the side that had been operated will often show higher amplitudes, mainly from faster rhythms, especially beta activity and at times alpha, too.[65] The effect of cutting the skull, regardless of what is done to the brain underneath, is to allow more fast activity to be recorded. Thus, the "abnormal" operated side will often show alpha of higher amplitude and the opposite side of *lower* amplitude will be the more normal side. Directions to technicians to seek out scalp scars reflecting previous craniotomies, in addition to complete histories, will help to avoid the trap of designating the lower amplitude alpha from the unoperated side as possibly an abnormal feature. The term *breech rhythm* is used to refer to these high amplitude rhythms, usually sharp in configuration, that can be recorded after the skull has been cut or "breeched."[66] The electroencephalographer should be cautious about call-

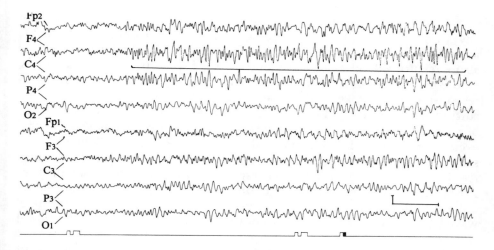

Figure 6.1 "Breech rhythm." Note Channel 2 (F4–C4), showing higher amplitudes and sharper rhythms over the area of a previous craniotomy.

ing all of these sharp rhythms "epileptiform" and should require that a single event be exquisitely paroxysmal before such a label is used (Fig. 6.1).

Slow Waves

General Comments

One of the major categories of EEG abnormality is the slow wave, referring to any wave slower than the expected normal pattern. Usually, theta (4 to <8 c/sec) and delta (<4 c/sec) waves, in addition to portions or pieces of slow waves, called *slow transients,* make up this category. Generally, these slow waves will appear in the waking record, frequently disappearing in the sleep tracing, and therefore (with rare exceptions) the EEG during the *waking state* without drowsiness is required to detect a slow wave abnormality.

A general understanding of slow waves and a simple neurophysiological mechanism as a way to view them may be helpful here. The brain waves that we record on the EEG are usually considered as spontaneously occurring, but some kind of driving stimulus or pacemaker can be hypothesized to exist. The frequency of these brain waves can be considered as reflecting the responsiveness of the neurones to that driving stimulus. In the case of alpha waves, the "stimulus" produces a quick response from the neural aggregates involved in this rhythm and in approximately 100 milliseconds (msec), those neurones have completely recovered from the previous response and are ready to respond again to the same constantly recurring pacemaker stimulus. Another rhythmical response occurs in the next 100 msec, and another, etc., so that a rhythmical alpha rhythm at 10 c/sec results, consisting of successive responses, each 100 msec in duration.

In the case of neurones that have been slightly damaged in some (or any) way, their responsiveness to some stimulus will be diminished and 200 msec (for example) may be required before those neurones can respond again, resulting in a 5 c/sec wave. In the case of severely damaged neurones, whose responsiveness has been greatly affected, a stimulus would produce a response that may take a full second of time before full recovery occurs, resulting in a waveform at 1 c/sec, a very slow delta wave. Thus, the frequency of a waveform can be properly viewed as reflecting its responsiveness or its excitability by the length of time taken to recover fully in readiness to respond again. Neural aggregates severely damaged by some type of pathology require long recovery periods after responding and are associated with very slow (delta) waves, while those with only a mild disturbance of function require shorter recovery periods or cycles and are associated with faster (theta) waves. See Figure 6.2 for examples of five different categories or degrees of slow wave abnormality that have been useful to this author.

Viewed in the context of recovery or excitability cycles, slow waves can be expected to be and are in fact only a *nonspecific* indication of a neurophysiological disturbance. Thus, they may not often point to a particular etiology, since any condition that renders neurones less excitable (hypoexcitable) can be associated with slow waves. But the distribution of the slow waves, their frequency, and occasionally other subtle features can suggest a certain given etiology, as is discussed below.

Diffuse

Diffuse vs. random

The diffuse appearance of slow waves, as expected, usually means that the brain has a *generalized* abnormality without any lateralization to one side or any focalization to any one area. The difference between diffuse slow waves seen randomly and random slow waves seen diffusely underscores one difficult problem that occasionally confronts the electroencephalographer. This problem is to determine which EEG patterns reflect truly a *diffuse* or generalized disturbance and which reflect a *deep* possibly focal *subcortical* midline disorder, projecting diffusely onto the cortex. In the first instance, *RANDOM* slow waves will be seen, referring to their appearance *HERE AND THERE* on *each and every area*, implicating each and every *CORTICAL* region. In the second instance, a given slow wave pattern will be seen *DIFFUSELY*, usually *SYNCHRONOUSLY AND SYMMETRICALLY* between the two sides, implicating a deep *SUBCORTICAL* origin projecting onto the cortex. The major point here is that each electroencephalographer should be aware of this difference and make clear in the report which condition applies. A clear separation of these two conditions is occasionally difficult, however, especially because both conditions often exist in the same patient. See Figures 6.3 and 6.4.

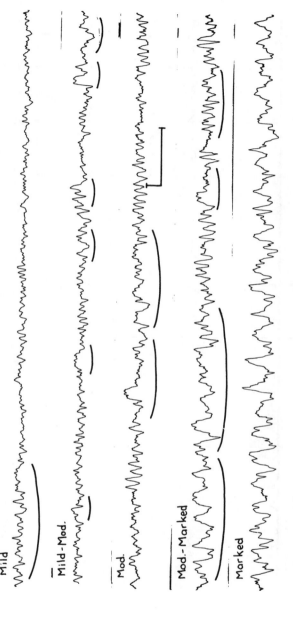

FIGURE 6.2   Various degrees of slow wave abnormalities. On top a mild degree is seen (a few slow transients), then below that a mild to moderate degree with considerable theta activity, a moderate with some delta waves, a moderate to marked with nearly 50% delta, and at the bottom a marked degree of slowing with nearly continuous delta waves.

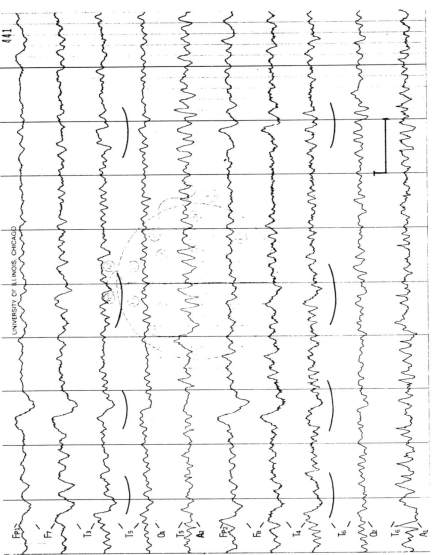

FIGURE 6.3   Diffuse slow waves. Note that the slowing (underlined) is usually seen diffusely on both sides, but appears symmetrical and synchronous, likely projected from subcortical regions.

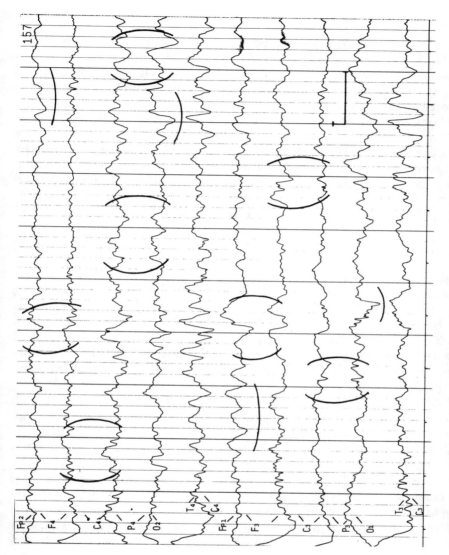

FIGURE 6.4   Random slow waves. Note that slow waves are seen from each and every region and are not synchronous on the two sides.

Associated medical conditions

A *DIFFUSE DISTURBANCE* can be expected, of course, in all those *CONDITIONS* that have a GENERALIZED effect on the brain. These conditions include metabolic, toxic, infectious, and also occasionally vascular and traumatic etiologies.[67] Since these latter conditions often affect midline subcortical nuclei as well, then symmetrical activity, simultaneously projected onto both sides, may also be found.[67] Truly FOCAL pathology, however, found *only* within the MIDLINE SUBCORTICAL structures and then appearing as *DIFFUSE* SYMMETRICAL ACTIVITY, can exist as a deep focus, especially a space-occupying lesion, including midline tumors, hemorrhages, etc. Diencephalic tumors tend to project maximally onto the frontal regions, and those in the posterior fossa region more often project on the occipital areas but also frontally to a lesser extent.[68]

Decreased frequency of background rhythm

Another form of a nonfocal abnormality is the decreased frequency of background rhythm, discussed here under the category of diffuse slow waves since the rhythms involved are abnormally slow and are nonfocal or diffuse. This background rhythm, usually within the alpha (8 to 13 c/sec) range in the older child and adult, can be considered as representing the general level of excitability within the central nervous system. When some condition slows down this level, the frequency of the background rhythm diminishes and the EEG should then be called abnormal.

ALL CONDITIONS THAT DIFFUSELY AFFECT THE BRAIN, such as metabolic, toxic, vascular, or infectious etiologies, can therefore be associated with a DECREASED FREQUENCY OF BACKGROUND RHYTHM,[67] in addition to significant focal pathology, which also involves subcortical regions and appears as projected slow waves. Abnormally slow background frequencies, however, are associated more often with some diffuse conditions than with others, especially METABOLIC disorders.[68] Hypothyroidism is an excellent example of a metabolic condition which usually changes this frequency, even to the point of correlating well with bone age, psychological test results sampling reactivity, and blood tests measuring thyroid function.[69,70,71] Improvement or deterioration in patients with cretinism or myxedema can often be properly assessed by plotting the changes in the frequency of the background rhythm.

Another condition usually associated with the slowing of the alpha is aging. Since *healthy* centenarians usually show background rhythms over 8 c/sec,[7,72] any decrease in frequency of the alpha in aged patients should remain above 8 c/sec. Background frequencies within the theta range (4 to < 8 c/sec) should be considered abnormal in the older age groups and will likely correlate with cognitive deficits beyond the norm for that particular age range.[73]

Focal

General comments

Pathology in *ANY* REGION of the brain, especially the cortex, from *ANY* ETIOLOGY can present with FOCAL SLOW WAVES, with degrees of severity ranging from VERY MILD TO VERY SEVERE. As previously indicated, these slow waves reflect a neurophysiological disturbance of those areas demonstrating the slowing and can arise from any etiology that focally disturbs the normal functioning of neurones. A slight concussion involving the left frontal area will likely show only a mild slow wave abnormality in that area, while a rapidly growing tumor of the same region would show a marked slowing. A second record later in time will show an improvement in the former and a deterioration in the latter instance. Some focal patterns require special comment, as noted below.

Frontal

Bilateral (1) Frontal intermittent rhythmic delta activity (FIRDA) or intermittent delta rhythms (IDR). See Figure 6.5.

As the first pattern to be discussed under the heading of *focal* slow waves, the FIRDA pattern is appropriate since it represents a link with the discussion of diffuse slow waves projected from subcortical regions (see under Diffuse, above). The major difference between the patterns just discussed and FIRDA is that the latter is *exclusively frontal, appears in organized repetitive bursts at a fixed frequency usually of 2.5 c/sec, is reactive to external stimuli, and is lost in sleep.*[68] This waveform indicates a neurophysiological disturbance within the *anterior brainstem structures,* especially the anterior diencephalon.[68] Any condition involving these subcortical gray structures can be associated with FIRDA, including deep midline tumors, metabolic conditions, especially diabetes mellitus, infectious and degenerative disorders (such as Heidenhain's encephalopathy), including neurometabolic errors in children (such as Batten's disease).[74] In contradistinction to FIRDA, another type of slowing is called *polymorphic delta activity,* which is nearly continuous, is nonreactive to stimuli, and reflects a white matter disturbance.

(2) Theta. Bilateral frontal slowing in the delta frequencies and appearing intermittently (FIRDA) has just been described; bifrontal activity in the theta range requires special comment. First, the differentiation of *abnormal* theta from *normal* patterns represents one of the most difficult problems in EEG. As was noted in the section on normal rhythms, the young child develops theta rhythms on the central (and frontal) regions as background rhythm and continues to show these rhythms even after the alpha develops on the occipital areas. As the posterior alpha further develops, the frontocentral theta diminishes, and the major problem for the electroencephalographer is to differentiate any of this (normal) remaining theta activity from

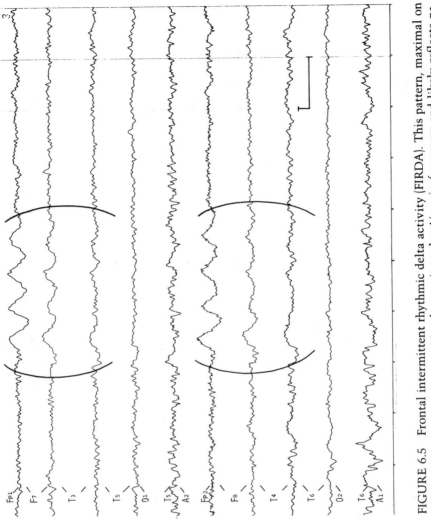

FIGURE 6.5 Frontal intermittent rhythmic delta activity (FIRDA). This pattern, maximal on the frontal areas, seen in repeating bursts, is under 4/sec in frequency and likely reflects pathology within near-midline, upper brain-stem, or diencephalic structures.

abnormal activity. Usually, the normal theta decreases in adolescence and disappears by late teens;[75] therefore, large amounts (higher in amplitude than alpha) in the teens or any significant amounts (>50μV) in the third decade can usually be considered abnormal. Another problem is to differentiate abnormal theta from similar activity that can appear in very early drowsiness. This latter activity can also represent a considerable problem for the electroencephalographer since it may be the only drowsy pattern to appear simultaneously with alpha activity, which usually designates a waking stage. Clearly, *normal frontal theta of drowsiness can be seen, while the alpha is present,* but its proper interpretation usually depends on other EEG signs of drowsiness that should appear within 5 to 10 seconds, such as the decrease in alpha. See Figure 6.6 for theta, related to drowsiness.

Abnormal frontal theta activity can therefore appear, especially in the second and third decades, as an exaggeration of activity that could be considered normal at an earlier age. One interpretation of this type of activity is that it represents a neurophysiological immaturity and some electroencephalographers have proposed that correlations can be found also for psychological immaturity.[76] *Organic lesions deep within the frontal areas, especially those that are subcortical near-midline within the diencephalic structures,* must be considered. Lesions around the third ventricle, including slow-growing space-occupying lesions, usually present electrographically as bifrontal theta rhythm.[68] Tumors within the same region that are rapidly expanding and other lesions associated with high rates of neuronal destruction usually show bifrontal *delta,* not *theta,* waves. See Figure 6.7 for an example of abnormally high amplitude theta waves.

Unilateral Unilateral frontal slow waves are seen whenever one frontal region includes neurones that are rendered hypoexcitable from some type of pathology. One particular etiology is frequently noted in EEG departments, and this refers to the CVA OR STROKE INVOLVING ONE CAROTID ARTERIAL SYSTEM. In this instance, the frontal area may show the maximal slow waves, but nearly an equal amount can be seen on the ipsilateral temporal area and the slowing can therefore be described as FRONTOTEMPORAL in locus. Frequently, however, the temporal area will show the most prominent slow waves. The locus of this slowing is reasonable and expected, especially in view of the distribution of the carotid artery, which feeds that same frontotemporal area. In many instances of carotid artery CVAs the contralateral side will show independent slowing, although no clinical findings may be evident that the other side is also involved. Thus, the EEG can be valuable in determining that a bilateral disturbance exists, although clinically only a unilateral lesion may be evident. THE DIFFERENTIATION BETWEEN A CVA AND A TUMOR MAY BE DIFFICULT; HOWEVER, REPEAT EEGs IN THE CVA USUALLY SHOW IMPROVEMENT AND IN THE TUMOR DETERIORATION.[68] IN ADDITION, TUMORS SHOULD BE CONSIDERED WHEN THE EEG IS MORE ABNORMAL THAN

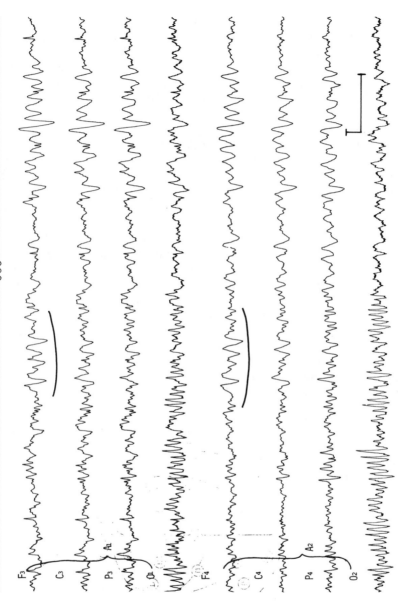

FIGURE 6.6   Frontal theta of drowsiness. Note on Channels 1 and 5 (frontal areas) the 5/sec theta rhythms while the *alpha* activity (Channel 4 and 8) *is present*. A few seconds later the drowsiness is revealed on *all* channels.

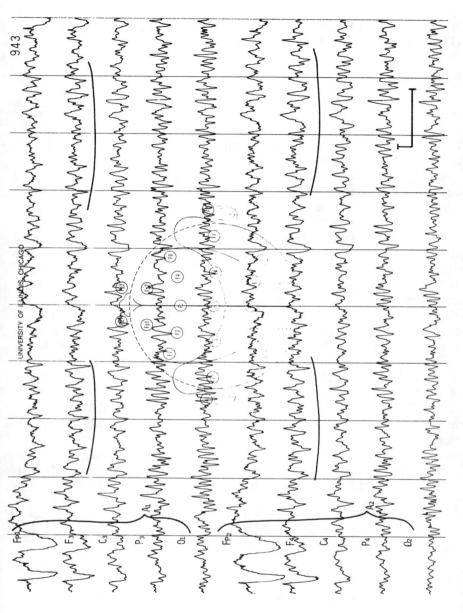

FIGURE 6.7 High amplitude frontal theta. Note Channels 2 and 6 from the frontal areas, showing theta waves at 4½ to 6½/sec, higher in amplitude than the alpha on Channels 5 and 10.

WOULD BE SUGGESTED BY THE CLINICAL PICTURE, ESPECIALLY
WITH POLYMORPHIC DELTA WAVES. SEE FIGURE 6.8.

Temporal

Temporal slow waves are the most common kind of EEG abnormality in the
majority of EEG laboratories. A number of reasons for this include the ex-
quisite sensitivity of neurones within the temporal lobe, especially of the
adult so that minor disturbances within the temporal lobe and even from
neighboring areas may show as temporal slowing.[77] Other reasons are that
the major pathological changes in aging, anoxic conditions, head injury and
many other etiologies are found *in* the temporal lobe,[78] especially within
the depth of this lobe, the amygdala and hippocampus. These disturbances
then present as slow wave abnormalities on the temporal lobe.

Temporal slowing during the aging process presents a definitional
problem of the term "normal." The *expected incidence* in percent of some
slow waves on the temporal lobe is approximately *one-half of the age*, so
that around 40% of all octogenarians will show some slowing.[79] If one defines normal only in terms of the statistical average for a given age group
without investigating various cognitive or motor deficits, then the designation of these slow waves (as long as they are not prominent delta waves) as
"normal" might seem justified, since nearly one-half of these individuals
show the slowing. On the other hand, if one defines normal in terms of the
healthy in that same age group, after having found no obvious cognitive or
motor deficit, then the designation of these slow waves as abnormal seems
justified. Thus, this problem of temporal lobe slowing is similar to the problem of the slowed frequency of the background rhythm. Although the statistical majority of aged individuals may show alpha <8 c/sec, *healthy*
centenarians show frequencies >8 c/sec. Similarly, the majority of the aged
may show some temporal slowing, but the *healthy* do not. One specific pattern called BORTT (bursts of rhythmical temporal theta)[80] is often seen as
a first sign of cognitive decline in these patients (see Fig. 6.9). Gibbs and
Gibbs[81] have referred to "minimal temporal slow activity" and Niedermeyer[82] has referred to "minor temporal slow" in similar conditions. Thus,
definite slow waves on the temporal lobe of aged patients, although common, can be called abnormal, often only mildly so. When appropriate tests
are run, such as a fluency test,[83] the appropriate electroclinical correlations
will often appear. Some investigators have failed to find any correlations
with these temporal slow waves, but others have found a relationship between only mild disturbances and a general cognitive deficit.[73] The prominence of *left*-sided temporal slowing is well known and often bitemporal
slow waves are more apparent on the *left* side.[70] This preference for the left
side may, in part, be related to the fact that the left temporal lobe involves
the speech area in most patients. Therefore, with left temporal slow waves
patients may seek medical attention more often than with right temporal

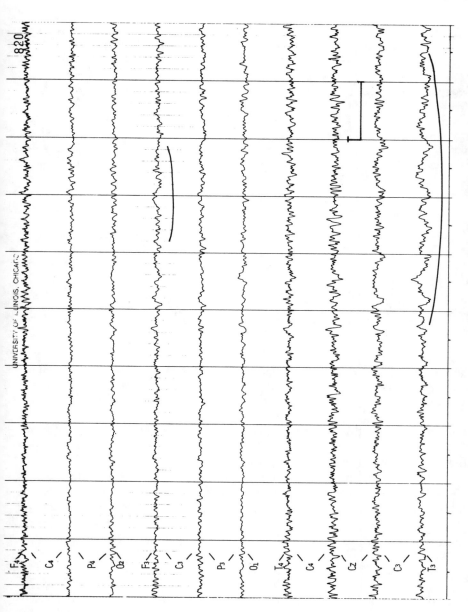

FIGURE 6.8   Slow waves on the left temporal area from a CVA. Note the last channel from the left temporal area, showing the slow waves, which occasionally spread to the left frontal area (Channel 4).

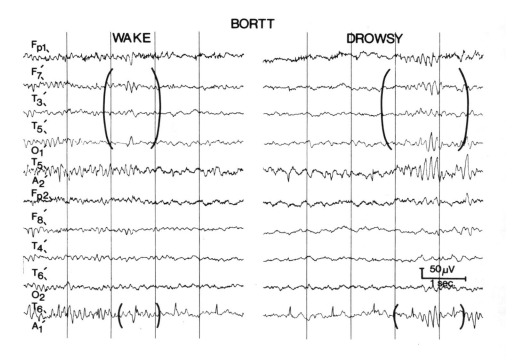

FIGURE 6.9   Burst of rhythmical temporal theta (BORTT). Note (left) the very short burst during wakefulness on Channels 2 to 4 (left temporal area), seen also on the last channel (left ear) and note also (right) the longer burst in the drowsy record.

slowing. However, this is only a partial explanation, since elderly individuals without obvious cerebral signs or symptoms, but with slow waves, also show a left temporal emphasis.[80,84] See Figure 6.10.

Temporal slowing is associated with *many different etiologies*, just as temporal pathology is found in most conditions that affect the brain. Since head injuries, regardless of site of impact, often involve the scraping of the temporal lobe along the inner part of the sharp, bony middle fossa, temporal slow waves are often seen following concussions or brain contusions.[85]

Parietal

The parietal areas seem somewhat special when slow waves are discussed. Their neurones seem relatively resistant to changes in excitability, in contrast to the temporal neurones, whose excitability is easily changed. Since the parietal region demonstrates this particular characteristic, certain conclusions follow. One conclusion is that delta rhythms are uncommon in this area, while *theta waves are more characteristic*,[86] as an example of a change in excitability that is only moderate (theta), rather than marked (delta). Another conclusion is that pathology located in the parietal areas, such as tu-

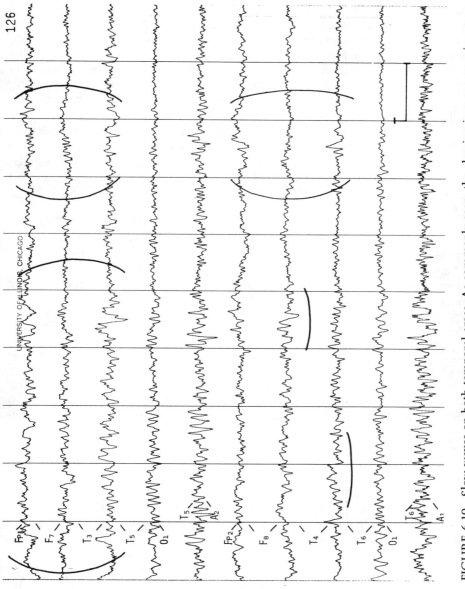

FIGURE 6.10 Slow waves on both temporal areas. As commonly seen, the slowing is more prominent on the left temporal area (first 5 channels) than the right (last 5 channels).

mors, are *more often missed or mislocalized* than for any other region.[87] Still another corollary may be that delta rhythms, *when they do occur* within the parietal areas, can be expected to reflect significant pathology, especially in adults. Since this region *usually* is not associated with any vascular etiologies, except for emboli, unilateral parietal slow waves, especially *delta rhythms in the adult,* should be considered as reflecting a *space-occupying lesion* until proven otherwise. The same conclusion applies to slow waves localized on the *central areas.*

Since parietal slow waves are often only theta in frequency, rather than delta, they may easily be missed. If the alpha frequency on the occipital areas is 8 to 8½ c/sec and the intermixed theta waves 6 to 7 c/sec, the nondiscriminating eye may not recognize the difference in these frequencies and see the parietal rhythms only as an extension of the occipital alpha. See Figure 6.11.

Parietal slow waves in the child likely have a *different significance* than in the adult. In the former instance these slow waves are usually an anterior extension of occipital slowing in the child, which is often *nonspecific* in character and discussed below. One author and his colleague[88] have suggested that parietal theta rhythms may, at times, indicate a genetic marker for primary generalized epilepsy.

Occipital

Children   Most normal children will show slow waves on the occipital areas until into the early twenties.[89] The *amount of slowing* will determine whether the record should be considered as abnormal. Pieces of slow waves, called "slow transients" by some electroencephalographers, are seen in these children, but should be decreasing in the mid-teens to nearly an absence in the early twenties. If these *transients continue in abundance, in the third decade, they may be considered abnormal,* representing a neurophysiological immaturity. Another form of occipital slowing, usually considered *abnormal,* is the *organized, rhythmical delta waves* (under 4 c/sec) that can be unilateral or bilateral.[89] These patterns should be considered *nonspecific,* since they have been described in some behavior and learning disorders, in addition to many other neurological conditions. See Figure 6.12.

Posterior fossa tumors. A specific category of occipital slowing consists of *low frequency irregular delta waves, at times symmetrical and at other times shifting* from one side to the other. These rhythms are usually projected from posterior fossa tumors, which are also associated from projected slow waves on the frontal regions as well, and at times diffusely.[90]

Adults   *Slow activity on the occipital areas,* usually in the form of slow transients rather than rhythmical slow waves, are seen in some adults who have *vascular disorders involving the vertebral-basilar system* or TIAs involving the posterior cerebral circulation.[91] In these same patients, *slow*

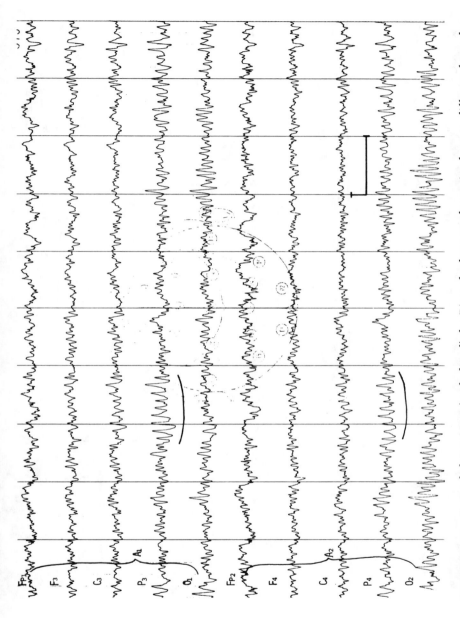

FIGURE 6.11 Parietal theta. Note (underlined) the 7/sec rhythms on the parietal areas, different from the alpha at 10–11/sec on the occipital areas.

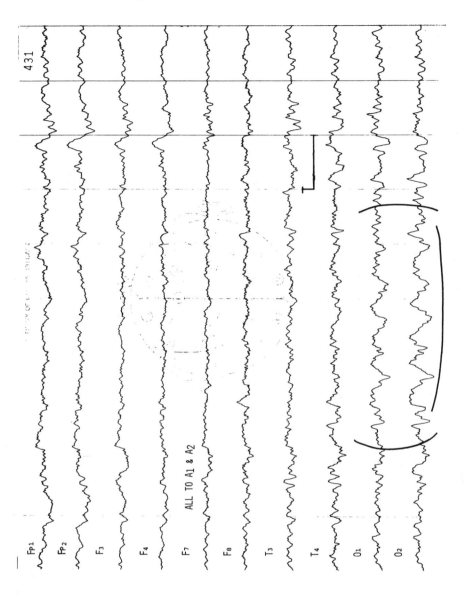

FIGURE 6.12　Excessive occipital slowing. Note on the last two channels the rhythmical delta waves of 1 and 2/sec.

waves on the temporal areas are also often seen, as might be expected in that the basilar artery bathes both the occipital area and certain portions of the temporal lobe.

Sharp Paroxysmal Activity

General Comments on Spikes, Spike and Wave Complexes, and Sharp Waves

Definitions

As previously indicated, the difference between the terms "spikes" and "sharp waves" is a matter of the duration of the discharge, whether less than 70 msec (spike) or between 70 to 200 msec (sharp wave),[1] and could be a reflection of the depth of the focus from the surface. The term *spike and wave complex* refers only to the presence of a prominent wave after each spike, likely reflecting the inhibitory processes after the excitatory spike.[92] The addition of the wave to the spike does not place this electrographic event into a different or special category, especially since some kind of wave can usually be seen after each spike or sharp wave, if filter settings permit them to be recorded. The addition of the wave is usually a reflection of a relatively active focus in the case of a *focal* spike and wave pattern, especially when the spike and wave complex repeats itself at a given frequency. Low amplitude spikes are usually associated with low amplitude waves that might easily be disregarded, while high amplitude spikes are usually seen with high amplitude waves. These latter complexes of high voltage are more often noted in patients with more active or severe forms of seizure disorder than the patients with relatively low amplitude paroxysmal activity. Thus, these three terms all refer to the same kind of paroxysmal activity, spikes possibly coming from more superficial foci than sharp waves[93] and spike and wave complexes showing with the wave the (deep) inhibitory hyperpolarizing processes after the spike.

The three overlapping characteristics for identifying a spike or sharp wave are its (1) paroxysmal character, (2) degree of sharpness, and (3) short duration. The most important is the paroxysmal aspect, namely, that the spike "shoots" suddenly out of the background rhythm. Although spikes from deep foci lose amplitude as they project toward the surface onto our electrodes, for a given depth *low* amplitude discharges likely come from *small* foci and *high* amplitude discharges arise from *large* foci. The low amplitude focus likely has only hundreds of neurones whose discharges are synchronized together, while the high amplitude focus has many thousands of synchronized neurones contributing to the discharge. The low amplitude spikes, like small sharp spikes, are well known to be associated less frequently with clinical seizures, compared to the high amplitude discharges; it makes intuitive sense that a large focus engaging many more neurones would have a greater probability of generating a clinical attack than a tiny focus with fewer neurones involved. Thus, in general, a *small* spike is often from a *small* focus with a *small* chance for a clinical seizure; a *large* spike is from a *large* focus with a *large* chance for a clinical attack.

Meaning and relationship to epilepsy

As long as an electroencephalographer properly identifies an abnormal, paroxysmal spike, spike and wave complex, or sharp wave, then a focus can be said to exist. The first problem, however, is to be certain that one is not misinterpreting normal events, such as the *vertex sharp transient*, which is also sharp and paroxysmal in character. The major difference between the two is that the *normal* vertex sharp *transient* is usually a broader, duller event with a wider distribution throughout the scalp, compared to the *abnormal* vertex sharp *wave* or spike that is sharper, more paroxysmal, and exquisitely focal. Various other potentials, such as the occipital lambda or the central mu rhythm, can be sharp in character, but the electroencephalographer must first properly identify the *abnormal* focus or diffuse discharge. The lambda wave is associated with eye movement and the mu waves arise from the C3,4 areas with alpha frequencies appearing in short or long bursts. If proper identification occurs, however, a focus then exists and in the case of the *diffuse* symmetrical spike and wave complex an entire neuronal network, the corticoreticular system, can be viewed as the origin of the epileptiform activity.

The next important issue is the clinical significance of such a focus. Clearly, *two kinds of events must occur for an epilepsy to exist in a patient.* First, there must be a *focus*, and second, it must *spread* its activity to manifest itself clinically. Some patients demonstrate on their EEG paroxysmal focal sharp waves and therefore can be said to have a focus, but have never had or may never have a clinical seizure, which likely depends on many factors, including an inherited threshold. Cortical areas vary considerably in the incidence of a clear seizure disorder associated with a focal discharge in that same area. For example, a spike or sharp wave on the frontal or central area is more often associated with clinical seizures than the occipital focus.[94] The latter focus is well known to exist in children who *may not* have clear seizures but who *may* have other clinical problems, for example, a visual perceptual disorder.[95]

Since both a focus and spread from the focus are required for a clinical seizure, it is therefore expected that all patients with spikes are not necessarily patients with epilepsy, i.e., he who spikes does not necessarily fit. On the other hand, such a patient has one of the two requirements for a seizure disorder and, although very controversial, more evidence is found to pay attention to these "asymptomatic" spikes.[96] By 1989 over 100 articles had been written about the effects of an interictal spike discharge on all of the different changes that can occur within the brain. In brief, nearly everything that happens in the brain, including neuronal, vascular, and metabolic changes, can be affected by the single interictal discharge.[97] Examples are that patients with occipital spikes respond late or not at all to a visual stimulus presented at the timing of the spike[98] or the driver of an automobile whose lateral movement on the road at the time of the discharge is abnormal, equivalent to the effects of a 5 mg dose of diazepam.[99] The mirror focus phenomenon[100] has been demonstrated at all levels of the evolutionary scale and this refers to the gradual formation of a focus on the opposite side of the brain from the original focus and foci can also develop on the same side,[101] likely from the constant firing of that original focus ipsilaterally. Thus, in time one focus may develop into two or more, possibly increasing the probability of a clinical seizure. In addition, some evidence exists that argues for cognitive, behavioral, or emotional disturbances associated with paroxysmal discharges,[102] but clearly this area is the most controversial in the field of EEG and epilepsy. The old adage of "treating only the patient and not the EEG," meaning that medication should be given only to those who have *clearly* demonstrated a definite clinical *seizure*, is not accepted by all. Some investigators[98] are beginning to view the single, interictal spike discharge as a "mini-seizure," since clear clinical and physiological changes can be demonstrated to occur at the time of some of these spikes. Some physicians with expertise in epilepsy and its "borderlands" have successfully used anticonvulsants in some patients with active foci and various cognitive, learning, behavioral, or emotional disorders *without* diagnosing these patients with epilepsy, a term reserved for those with clear seizures.

Interictal and ictal activity (see Figs. 6.13, 6.14)

In the great majority of instances when the EEG confirms an epilepsy in a given patient, the EEG shows *interictal* (between seizures) rather than ictal (during seizure) activity. THE INTERICTAL EVENT IS IN THE FORM OF A SPIKE, SPIKE AND WAVE COMPLEX, OR SHARP WAVE DISCHARGE, SIGNALING THE PRESENCE OF A FOCUS. At the moment that the single, isolated spike fires, the brain is *not* in a clinical seizure but is only announcing the presence of a focus. When a CLINICAL SEIZURE OCCURS, VERY DIFFERENT ACTIVITY IS SEEN IN THE EEG DURING THIS *ICTAL* PERIOD, CONSISTING USUALLY OF *RHYTHMICAL* WAVEFORMS, as opposed to the interictal single isolated spikes. The relationship of the single interictal spike to the very different rhythmical ictal waveform is much like the relationship of the ticking of a time-bomb to the explosion from it. The ticking signals the presence of the device which may not explode, depending on various factors in the same way that the spike indicates a focus that may or may not "explode" in the form of a clinical seizure, depending on various other factors.

Ictal activity is nearly always recorded on the EEG when the seizure itself occurs during the recording, providing definite evidence for an

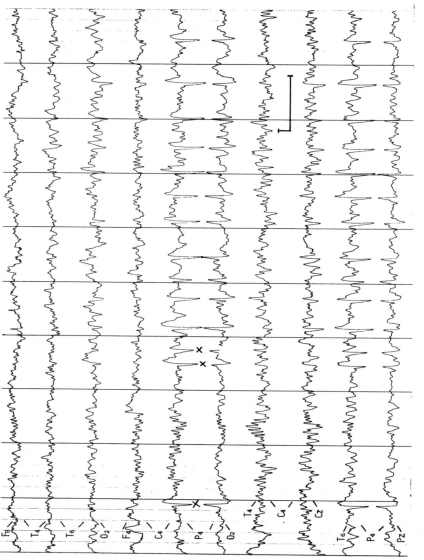

FIGURE 6.13   Sharp waves, as an interictal event. These discharges signal the presence of a focus, seen here on the right parietal (P4) area. Note the phase reversals between Channels 5 and 6 and also 9 and 10.

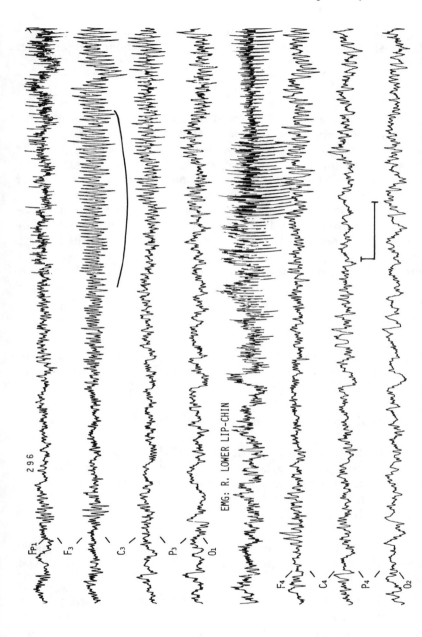

FIGURE 6.14 Focal ictal rhythms associated with focal clinical seizure. On Channel 2 note the rhythmical fast activity from 25→16/sec (left frontocentral area) associated in time with the muscle artifact on Channel 5 resulting from the (ictal) jerking of the right lower lip and chin. The seizure activity in the EEG seems to have a one-to-one relationship with the peripheral expression of the seizure in the form of muscle jerks.

epilepsy. Since the EEG more often records interictal events, however, most of the EEG classifications of the epilepsies are based on the interictal rather than ictal EEG.

Ontogenetic Approach

Most electroencephalographers understand that age plays a very important role in (1) the type of seizure disorder manifested by individuals and also (2) the type of EEG discharge shown by these patients. In other words, given the *age of a person with epilepsy, the kind of seizure disorder and its interictal EEG expression can often be predicted.* This prediction is possible since each age range seems to be associated with certain neuronal networks or cortical areas that have the greatest predisposition for developing a discharge. With maturation of the brain, various areas or networks become the primary target or most likely focus. Thus, given the age of the patient, the kind of EEG discharge (and clinical seizure) can often be predicted. In the following EEG classification of the epilepsies, which has a close correspondence to the clinical classification of the seizure disorders, such an ontogenetic approach will be presented.

Neonatal patterns

The first general point is that the best prognostic value for an EEG in the neonate is during the first five days of life past term.[31] Poor prognosis can be predicted under certain conditions. They are:

1. Low amplitude, less than 15 μV, or slow delta waves in the waking record.[103]
2. Low amplitude, less than 25 μV, in quiet (NREM) sleep.[31]
3. The absence of lability, spatial organization, or synchrony.[104]
4. Low voltage background and high voltage sharp waves or spikes.[31]
5. Positive central and temporal sharp waves.[105]
6. Dissociated clinical and EEG seizures.[106]

The reader will note that the last three features with poor prognosis relate to epileptiform activity, appropriate here since this section deals specifically with seizure patterns.

Positive Central and Temporal Sharp Waves   Single positive sharp waves (see Fig. 6.15) often may look like electrode artifacts, since we often see positive deflections as nonbrain activity. These positive discharges, not uncommon in the infant, can also be very focal as if from *only one* electrode, thereby leaving the further impression of artifacts. These sharp waves have often been associated with *intraventricular hemorrhage,*[105] the first etiology that one should consider, but they are not pathognomonic of such an etiology. The earlier descriptions of the neonatal positive sharp wave placed

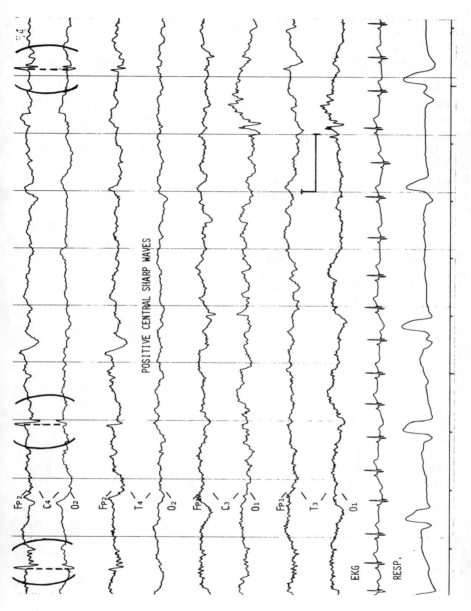

FIGURE 6.15   Positive central sharp waves. Note the separation of pens 1 and 2, indicating a prominent positivity in the discharge from the C₄ electrode.

them on the central areas, but more recently the same kind of discharges have been described on the temporal areas,[107,108] where they may be seen more often (>2:1).[107] They are usually associated with periventricular leukomalacia, intraventricular hemorrhage, infarcts,[108] and at times (29%)[107] with seizures.

Dissociated Clinical and EEG Seizures   Either a clinical epileptic attack that does not have EEG representation or an electrographic seizure without clinical manifestations is associated with a poor prognosis.[106] Figure 6.16 shows the beginning of an electrographic seizure without clinical manifestations and demonstrates an ictal pattern in the theta (5 c/sec) range. For contrast, Figure 6.17 shows another frequency, namely beta rhythms at 18 c/sec, as an ictal activation. Thus, fast or slow rhythms (or medium frequencies) may appear as ictal patterns. This dissociation introduces a very important point representing a "revolution" in pediatric epileptology. Two kinds of seizures are now described in the neonate: (1) those with EEG confirmation showing ictal rhythms and therefore called "epileptic seizures" and (2) those without EEG confirmation and called "nonepileptic seizures."[109] The epileptic type is *usually* associated with *focal* tonic or clonic seizures and the nonepileptic type with *generalized* tonic posturing or motor automatisms. The *nonepileptic* type could represent either brain stem release phenomena or subcortical epileptic activity not seen by our scalp electrodes.

Multifocal Independent Foci   As seen in Figure 6.18, *foci that are multifocal and independent are not uncommon in the neonate.* The multiplicity of these foci is much more common in the neonate and young infants than in the older ages. The periodicity of these discharges on the *temporal* areas, as seen in this figure, is very suggestive of *herpes simplex encephalitis*, not only in the infant but also at any age through adulthood. In Figure 6.19, some bilaterally synchronous discharges are noted in addition to the focal ones, but the former is uncommon in prematures and neonates.

Clonic Seizure and Typical Electrographic Correlate   Figure 6.20 shows an EEG of a neonate in a *clonic seizure* and shows a typical pattern often seen during this type of seizure, namely, a *repetitive spike discharge,*[110] occurring at the time of the clinical seizure. This kind of electrographic pattern as a long burst of focal spike or spike and wave complexes, is not seen as often in older patients who more often show organized *rhythms* as their ictal activity.

Tonic Seizure and Typical Electrographic Pattern   Figure 6.21 shows an EEG with a *slow delta discharge,* typical of the usual pattern seen during a *tonic* attack in the neonate.[110]

Harmonic Ictal Patterns   Figure 6.22 shows single repetitive discharges on the right temporal area as an interictal pattern and Figure 6.23 demonstrates

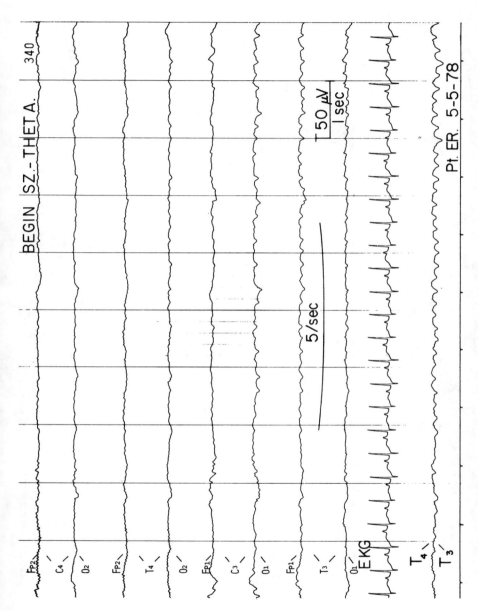

FIGURE 6.16 Beginning of electrographic seizure. Note the 5/sec rhythms, especially on Channel 7.

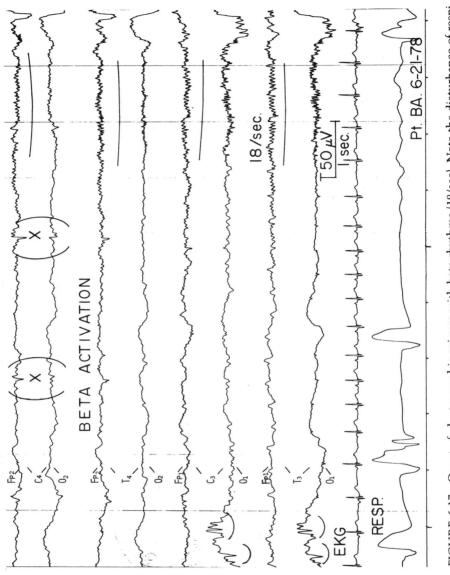

FIGURE 6.17 Onset of electrographic seizure with beta rhythms (18/sec). Note the disturbance of respiration (last channel).

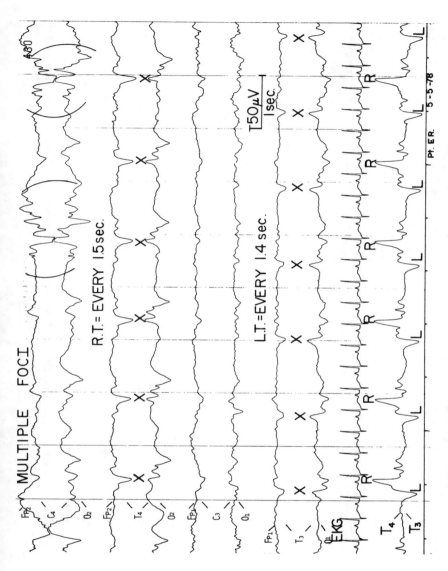

FIGURE 6.18 Multi-focal independent foci. Note the discharges on the right temporal area every 1.5 seconds and on the left temporal every 1.4 seconds. Sharp events are also seen from the C_4 electrodes.

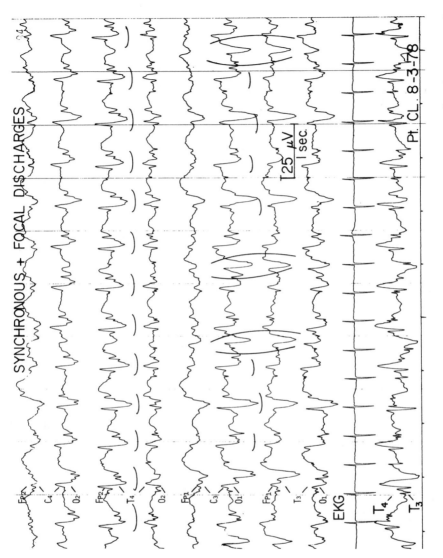

FIGURE 6.19   Synchronous and also focal discharges. The underlined portions reflect (uncommon) synchronous activity, but interspersed are some (more common) focal discharges, noted in brackets.

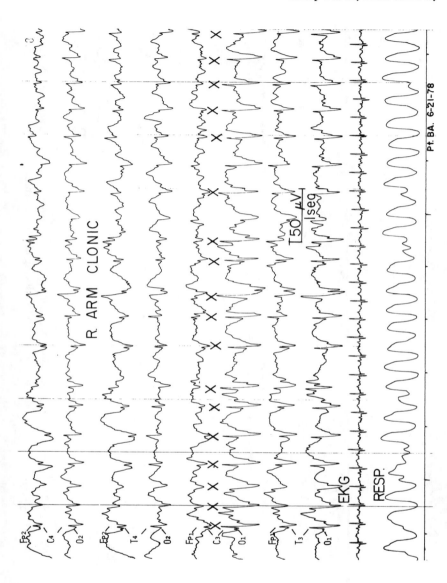

FIGURE 6.20 Characteristic repetitive discharge with clonic seizure. Right arm was seen in a clonic attack while the left central area showed a repetitive discharge at 1–2/sec.

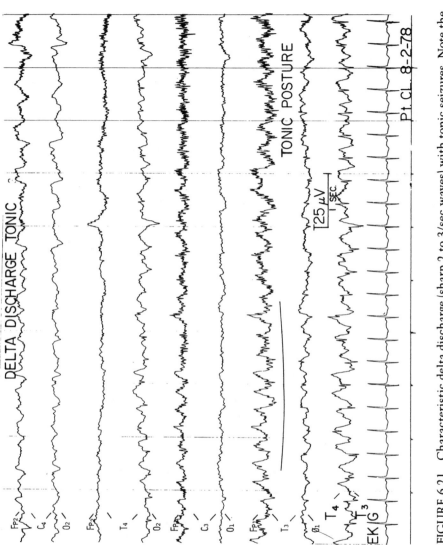

FIGURE 6.21   Characteristic delta discharge (sharp 2 to 3/sec waves) with tonic seizures. Note the muscle artifact, especially on Channels 5 and 7, during the tonic attack.

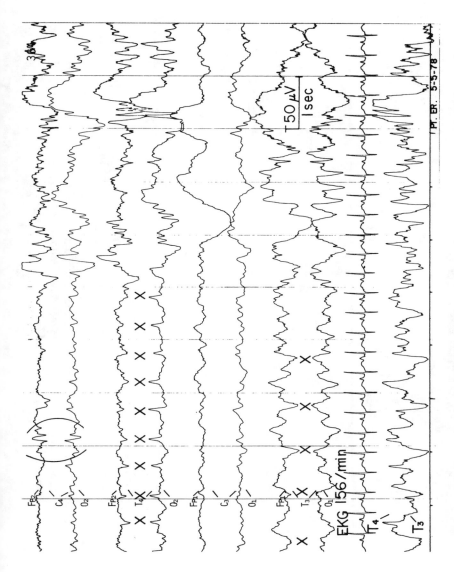

FIGURE 6.22 Repetitive discharge on right temporal area. Also note less prominent activity of a similar type from the left temporal and right central area.

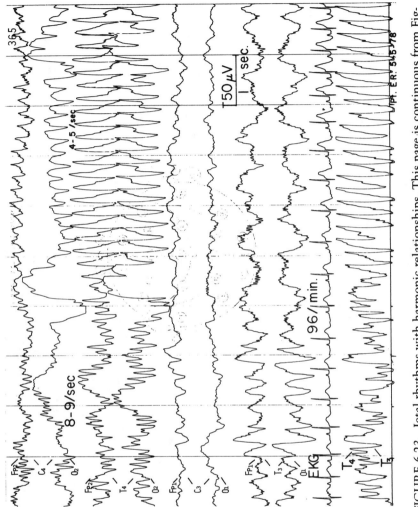

FIGURE 6.23 Ictal rhythms with harmonic relationships. This page is continuous from Figure 6.22 and shows rhythmical 8 to 9/sec waves, followed by 4 to 5/sec waves, as ictal rhythms, seen especially on Channels 3 and 4.

clear ictal rhythms at 9/sec on that same region and also at the subharmonic at 4 to 5 c/sec during a clinical seizure. *Harmonic or subharmonic relationships* (2 to 4 times or $\frac{1}{2}$ to $\frac{1}{4}$ the fundamental frequency) of *ictal patterns* are not only commonly seen in *neonates*, but *appear at all ages*. It is important to add that the brain talks to us with harmonic and subharmonic frequencies, not only in abnormal, but also in normal rhythms. Thus, there are 3 c/sec, 6 c/sec, and 12 c/sec (bilateral) spike and wave complexes, 6 to 7 and 14 c/sec positive spikes, 5 to 6 and 10 to 12 c/sec rhythmic mid-temporal discharges and also alpha variant at 5 and 10 c/sec, photic driving responses at harmonics and subharmonics, etc.

Theta pointu alternant[111]—5th day seizures[112]

The EEG pattern, called "theta pointu alternant," consists of alternating sharp activity at a theta frequency during an interictal period. This pattern can be seen in 60% of patients with 5th day seizures, occurring usually on the 5th day of life (after term), also called "benign idiopathic neonatal convulsions."[89] The seizures, lasting 1 to 3 minutes, are usually clonic or apneic, but not tonic, in an infant who is normal before and after the seizure.

Suppression burst—early infantile epileptic encephalopathy (EIEE) (see Fig. 5.11)

The suppression burst pattern, also called *burst suppression*, is characteristic of pathological coma at any age, but also is a distinctive pattern for EIEE,[113] appearing in infants at about 1 month of age with tonic spasms, often with brain malformations. The same EEG pattern, suppression burst, is seen in a related condition, called *neonatal myoclonic encephalopathy*.[114] This related condition is characterized more by massive myoclonus with a genetic component. In 6 months nearly half of these infants will die and survivors will often later show hypsarrhythmia.

Hypsarrhythmia—infantile spasms (see Fig. 6.24)

The term *hypsarrhythmia* means high or lofty arrhythmia, can be viewed as "mass chaos" on the EEG, and represents a severe form of a seizure disorder. Typically, patients first show this pattern at 4 to 6 months of age at a time when *infantile spasms* (often when mental and physical retardation) appear as the usual clinical manifestation of this activity. This type of seizure is characterized by lightning-like, brief extensor (cheerleader) or flexor (jackknife) spasms, often seen with head-nodding, and therefore also called Salaam seizures. The *hypsarrhythmic* pattern (as interictal activity) refers essentially to the presence of *paroxysmal sharp waves*, spikes, or spike and wave complexes seen independently on *all cortical regions*, in addition to a *diffuse slow wave abnormality on a poorly organized or non-existent*

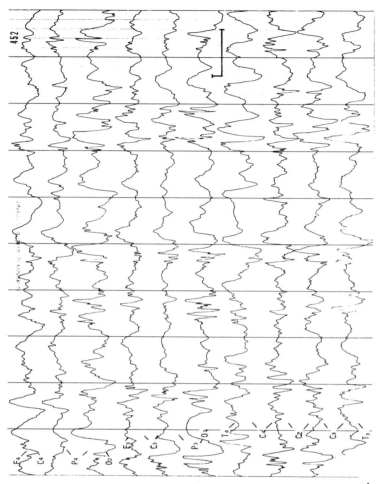

FIGURE 6.24   A. Hypsarrhythmia. This pattern is characterized by many sharp waves or spikes on each area (each channel), diffuse slow waves of high amplitude, and poorly organized background rhythm, seen between attacks. *B.* During the attack, called an *infantile spasm,* the diffuse discharges and high amplitude slow waves disappear (electrodecremental seizure), but questionable fast activity (Channel 6) can sometimes appear as a possible correlate of the clinical attack.

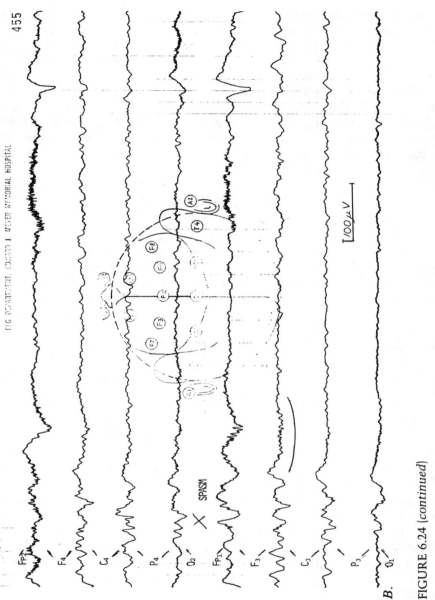

FIGURE 6.24 (continued)

background rhythm.[94] The ictal EEG (*during* the seizure) appears very different from the hypsarrhythmia and usually shows only low amplitudes (electrodecremental seizure),[115] but close inspection frequently reveals low voltage fast rhythms that likely represent ictal (seizure) activity. Other ictal patterns that can appear include generalized spike and wave complexes, high voltage slow rhythms on the frontal areas, or diffuse alpha or beta frequencies. The medication of choice is ACTH;[116] clonopin can also be helpful.[117] In the new classification of generalized epilepsies and syndromes[118] these seizures are considered Cryptogenic or Symptomatic–West Syndrome. West refers to an English physician who described these seizures in his own son in 1841.[119]

Slow spike and wave complexes—Lennox-Gastaut Syndrome[120,121] *(see Fig. 6.25)*

As the brain matures, the commissural systems that tie together the two halves of the brain begin to be more functional and synchronous and symmetrical activity from the two sides appear more frequently. At the end of the first year of life the patient with hypsarrhythmia usually shows less independent activity from the many foci on both sides and more synchronous patterns, usually in the form of spike and wave complexes. These complexes are similar to the pattern seen in "petit mal" epilepsy, so Frederic Gibbs[94] called them "petit mal variant," the latter term added since the frequency of the spike and wave was 1 to 2/sec, rather than 3/sec as in the classical "petit mal" pattern. In addition, the "petit mal variant" usually shows some degree of asymmetry and asynchrony. Patients with this waveform are generally 1 to 4 years of age, either developing it from hypsarrhythmia or beginning their seizure disorder anew with this waveform.

Clinical attacks are usually *generalized*, often *tonic* in character,[122] but atypical absence, clonic, atonic, or myoclonic attacks can also occur with physical and especially mental retardation as typical features. This condition can be considered the most severe form of epilepsy. The syndrome is named for two other investigators who studied the condition, Dr. William Lennox (U.S.A.) and Dr. Henri Gastaut (France). Benzodiazepines (Klonopin and Valium) are often used as anticonvulsants for this condition,[123] but Clobazam, available in Europe and Canada, has been the most successful.[124] A new anticonvulsant released in 1993, called Felbamate, also has promise.[125]

Bilateral 3/sec spike and wave complexes— corticoreticular seizures (see Fig. 6.26)

Bilaterally synchronous and symmetrical 3/sec spike and wave complexes appear in patients who have "petit mal" attacks. This latter term has been used in many different ways, often referring to any *small* or minor attack, so the term has been replaced in the new International Classification of Seizures by the term "absence." This term essentially describes the nature of

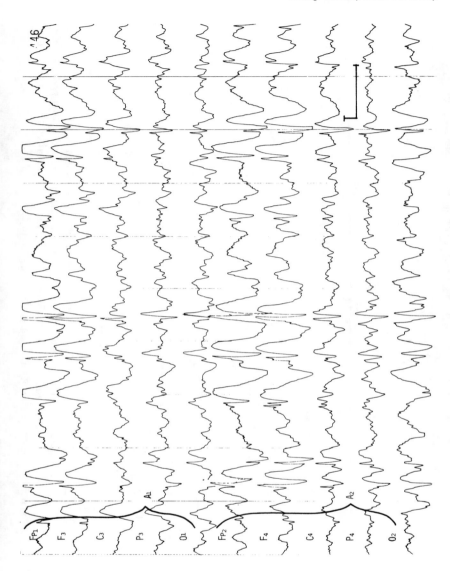

FIGURE 6.25   Lennox-Gastaut Syndrome (petit mal variant). Note the bilateral spike and wave complexes at a very slow repetition rate (1½ to 2/sec) with various degrees of shifting asymmetry.

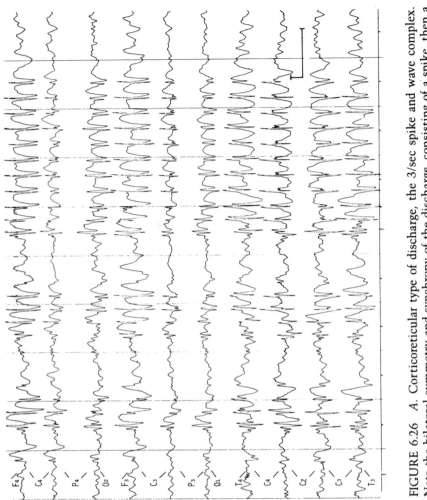

FIGURE 6.26 *A.* Corticoreticular type of discharge, the 3/sec spike and wave complex. Note the bilateral symmetry and synchrony of the discharge, consisting of a spike, then a wave, with the repetition frequency of 3/sec. This discharge is also called a primary bilateral synchrony. (See following pages for parts *B, C, D,* and *E.*)

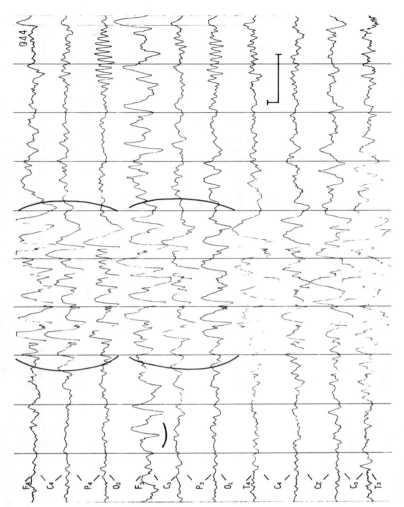

FIGURE 6.26 *B.* Secondary bilateral synchrony. In contrast with (A), these bilateral spike and wave complexes are initiated by a unilateral focal discharge (see Channel 4 from the left frontal area), then activating midline structures, which then project bilaterally synchronous complexes to both sides.

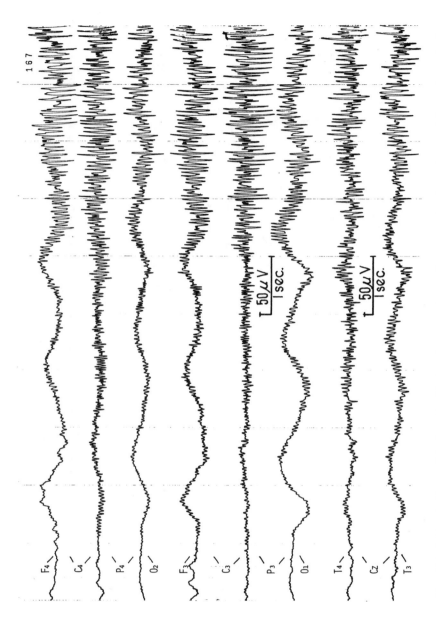

FIGURE 6.26   *C.* Generalized tonic-clonic seizure, at times also appearing in patients with corticoreticular seizure disorders. Onset of this seizure is indicated by diffuse fast activity at 18 to 20/sec, increasing in amplitude with time.

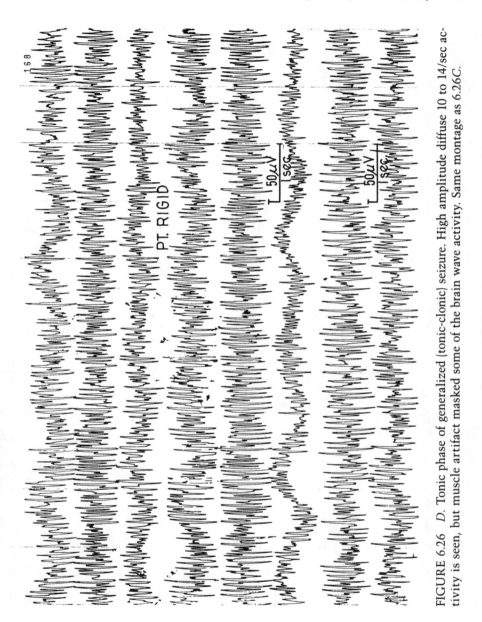

FIGURE 6.26 *D.* Tonic phase of generalized (tonic-clonic) seizure. High amplitude diffuse 10 to 14/sec activity is seen, but muscle artifact masked some of the brain wave activity. Same montage as 6.26*C.*

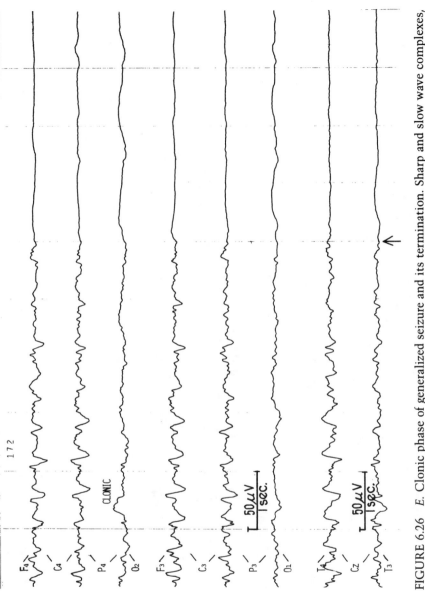

FIGURE 6.26   *E.* Clonic phase of generalized seizure and its termination. Sharp and slow wave complexes, seen diffusely, are noted with each clonic jerk and suddenly the seizure terminates (arrow). After the seizure, very depressed activity and (postictal) slow waves appear on both sides.

the attacks of these patients who have episodes (often 4 to 6 seconds in duration) of *staring or inattention*, usually with *eyelid fluttering* and frequently accompanied by *automatisms*, such as picking at the clothes, clearing of the throat, and various mouth movements. The EEG at the time of the spell shows the *3/sec spike and wave complexes*, which can also be short-lasting, for 1 second or so. Careful investigation into the clinical correlations of these spike and wave complexes indicates that as early as 0.5 seconds after their onset the majority of patients will show inattention,[126] suggesting that *very short-lasting spells of a second or less may have a cognitive effect on the patient*. Since these complexes do not cause unconsciousness, but only staring or inattention, some patients have been able to function intellectually to some limited degree during these episodes. For example, some patients can count forward but not backward and can answer simple, but not complex, questions during their attacks. Other patients, however, can answer no questions during an absence. Since the relationship of these attacks to awareness should not be considered all-or-none, but instead demonstrates *varying degrees of gradation*, the concept of "neural noise" can be useful in this context. Thus, the bilateral spike and wave complexes are a direct reflection of neural noise imposed into the cognitive system that makes difficult the receiving of any stimulus or signal. At times, the signal is strong enough to overcome the noise and no clear clinical effects may then be seen, but at other times the noise overwhelms all signals and the patient can only stare and cannot respond to any stimulus.

Since the essence of these attacks was a change in awareness, the major function of the subcortical reticular activating system (which was really equivalent to the "centrencephalon" of Penfield and Jasper),[127] the attacks and the associated EEG pattern were called "centrencephalic." Considerable research by Gloor,[128] however, has shown that the *cortex is more involved than the reticular system*, so the new term for these complexes is *corticoreticular*. Since the cortex seems to have a primary involvement in this disorder, it is not surprising that the EEGs of these patients often show discrete spike foci "here and there, now and then." Only if a given focus repeatedly appears in a tracing, otherwise with bilaterally synchronous spike and wave complexes, should such a focus be considered significant and reported as separate from the bilateral complexes.

The age of patients with 3/sec spike and wave complexes is often around 6 or 14 years, rarely appearing first before 3 or after 16 years of age.[94] In females, attacks often accompany the onset of menses at approximately 13 to 14 years.

In addition to the staring spells or absences, two other clinical forms, commonly associated with 3/sec spike and wave complexes, are the *myoclonic and akinetic* (now more properly called atonic) attacks, constituting the "petit mal triad" of William Lennox.[120] In the former, short-lasting bilateral jerks, especially of the arms, and in the latter a sudden loss of motor tone, accompany the spike and wave complexes, which usually differ from those of the absence by being *more irregular, shorter-lasting duration, often with poly- or multiple spikes with each wave.*[129] *If multiple spikes* are seen in the *waking* record of a patient with absence attacks, this EEG finding often foretells that *generalized tonic-clonic* attacks may also occur.[130] In 37% of these patients, evidence can be found of an inheritance factor[131] but more recent data indicate that at age 7 to 14 years as many as 88% of siblings to those with clear clinical attacks will show the signature of some bilateral spike and wave complexes in their EEG, especially in the sleep record.[132]

Depakene or Depakote is a very useful anticonvulsant for both the absence and the associated generalized tonic-clonic attacks.[132] Zarontin handles the absence part of the clinical attacks, but the addition of other drugs such as Dilantin is often required if generalized attacks occur as well.[133] A number of studies have shown that Tegretol can aggravate these complexes and therefore should not be used in cases of absences.[134] For the myoclonic and atonic types, clonopin is often very helpful.[135]

Occipital sharp waves—benign occipital epilepsy
(see Fig. 6.27)

These sharp waves on the most posterior of electrodes are usually seen in *preadolescent children,*[94] and if they are found in the adult, a space-occupying lesion should be considered. In the child they may relate to a *visual disorder,* for example, a visual perceptual or oculomotor disorder[95] and in patients with a complete retrolental fibroplasia,[136] virtually all these children can be expected to develop occipital discharges. This development is likely one of nature's unfortunate experiments demonstrating the hyperexcitability (spikes and sharp waves) from a denervation, that is, loss of afferent activity to the occipital areas as a result of a damaged retina. The fact that most of these children will not have clear clinical seizures emphasizes one feature of the occipital discharge, that *definite seizures are often not found.*[94] Attacks, however, may occur and do involve some visual experience in approximately 67% of those with some type of seizure. The remaining patients with this focus who have attacks show *clinical features according to which area receives the spread of epileptiform activity.*[137] Thus, a psychomotor attack may result from a spread from the occipital area to the temporal region or a focal motor attack if spreading to the sensorimotor cortex. Most of the children (92%) with these discharges and also clinical attacks will be free of seizures by their teens after appropriate anticonvulsant treatment. Therefore, Gastaut has called this syndrome "benign occipital epilepsy"[138] and has also pointed out that the condition has a relationship to basilar migraine, since symptoms such as headaches and nausea often occurring at the end of these attacks are suggestive of this type of migraine.

In patients with definite seizures the usefulness of Dilantin or Tegretol should be considered.[94]

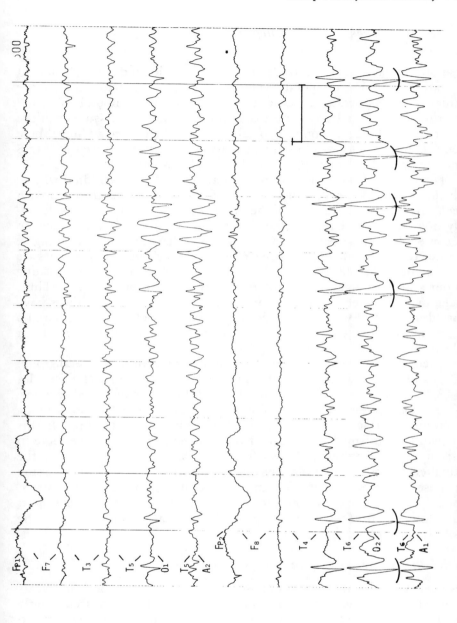

FIGURE 6.27 Occipital sharp waves. Note these sharp waves on Channel 9 from the right occipital areas, seen spreading to the left side (Channel 4).

Central sharp waves—benign epilepsy of childhood[139-143] (see Fig. 6.28)

These sharp waves are localized on the central electrodes (C3,4), but at times are close to the temporal electrodes (T3,4), and therefore the seizure disorder that is associated is sometimes called "centro-temporal epilepsy." Since the foci are usually very near the central or Rolandic fissure (over the "motor strip") the condition is also called "Rolandic epilepsy." Since there is remission in most cases by 9 to 12 years of age, after an onset at 5 to 8 years, the name "benign epilepsy of childhood" also applies.

The nature of the attacks in more than 50% of these children will be in the form of a *nocturnal motor attack, often as a hemifacial spasm with speech arrest*. Since both sides of the brain are often involved, the side initially involved may change in the next attack. Inherited factors appear to play some role in these patients. As many as 55% have attacks only at night, and since they do not *usually* involve noisy, violent movements, parents are not awakened; the child falls back to sleep and awakens in the morning without a bitten tongue and without urinary or fecal incontinence. Thus, attacks may be unrecognized for some time. However, some authors have reported up to 20% who also have generalized tonic-clonic seizures and a few are not benign, since they are not easily stopped with anticonvulsant medication such as Dilantin or Tegretol.

A recent study[144] has identified two different foci in this general group: (1) C3,4 and (2) C5,6 areas more lateral to C3,4 between the latter electrodes and T3,4. The C3,4 foci were seen in 31% and this group had focal seizures. The C5,6 foci were seen in 69% of patients who specifically had drooling and oromotor attacks, and also generalized tonic-clonic seizures. If this study can be confirmed, the benign nature of the disorder may be more in question. Also the presence of these foci on an EEG, often very active in the waking record and without obvious clinical attacks, has left the impression that these active discharging foci may be, at times, only EEG curiosities, especially when no one is monitoring whether attacks are occurring at night. Patients with these foci need more than casual investigation into the possibility of nocturnal seizures.

Parietal sharp waves—versive or sensory seizures

These discharges[145] are uncommon, but have an onset age of 4 to 8 years (3:1 male); clear clinical seizures associated with the focus are seen in only 25% of those with such a focus. Of those with clinical attacks, 75% are versive (turning away from the side with the focus), 10% have generalized tonic-clonic attacks, and some have sensory seizures. Slightly over 40% have a history of previous febrile seizures. One distinctive feature in this disorder is that these spikes may be elicited by taps on the heal as a kind of "reflexive discharge," representing a very excitable parietal region. Four

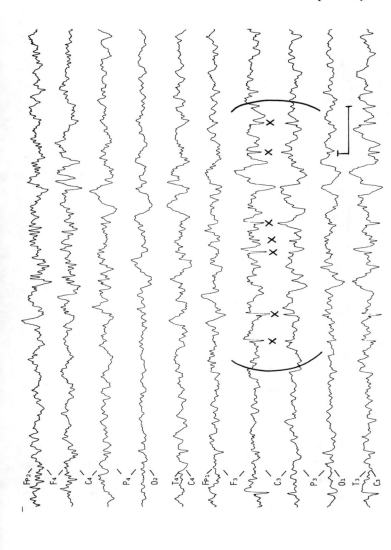

FIGURE 6.28   Central (and temporal) sharp waves. These sharp waves are seen on the left central area (Channels 7, 8) and are also well represented on the mid-temporal area. In this instance (a child of 8 years) note that the sharp wave does not spread well to adjacent channels (e.g., to Channel 6 from the left frontal area). This tendency of discharges to appear only on a given area without spreading to nearby electrodes is seen more often in children than in adults.

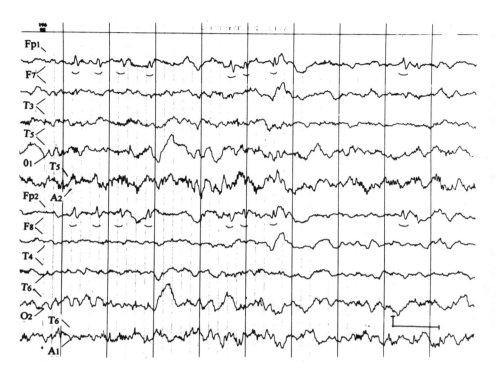

FIGURE 6.29   Prefrontal sharp waves. Note the many sharp waves (underlined) on Channels 1 and 6 from the prefrontal areas, often synchronous and symmetrical, likely arising from (deep) orbital frontal regions. Age, 5 years.

phases can at times be identified: (1) spikes only in the somatosensory evoked potential, (2) spikes in the sleep EEG, (3) spikes also in the wake EEG, and (4) clinical seizures. Nearly 100% of these patients with appropriate anticonvulsant drugs are seizure free by 12 years of age. Patients without seizures are often referred for an EEG because of learning or behavioral disorders.

Prefrontal sharp waves—neurovegetative seizures

These discharges (see Fig. 6.29) are uncommon, but likely arise from orbital frontal regions. This latter region is neuroanatomically connected via the uncinate fasciculus to the anterior temporal lobe and the clinical manifestations are therefore neurovegetative in type, always suggestive of a temporal lobe phenomenon. The seizures, arising in children 6 to 12 years of age, are often seen in clusters (up to 50/day), with a mean duration of 25 seconds, especially at sleep onset, including facial flushing; mydriasis; piloerection; abdominal complaints, such as butterflies or pain; fear; vocalization (screaming); but also repetitive movements.[146]

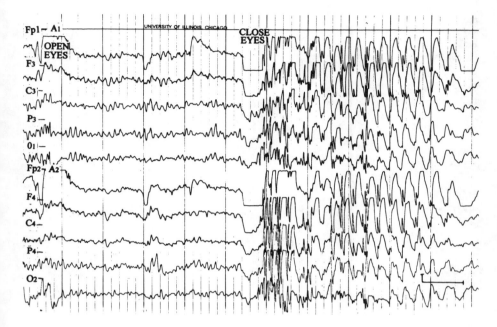

FIGURE 6.30   Bilateral spike and wave complexes elicited by eye closure, usually associated with bioccipital spike and wave complexes. Although the complexes seen here were at first generalized and later in this burst were maximal on the frontal areas, the majority throughout the rest of the record were bioccipital spike and wave complexes.

Bioccipital spike and wave complexes—partial
and generalized seizures

Earlier sections have discussed bilateral spike and wave complexes of a corticoreticular or generalized type and also focal occipital spikes or sharp waves. Occasionally patients may show a combination of these two patterns as bilaterally synchronous spike and wave complexes, maximal on the occipital areas, often noted immediately after eye-closure[147] (see Fig. 6.30). As might be expected patients may show aspects both of the (1) generalized corticoreticular form by their absences and also of the (2) focal occipital form by partial seizures, migraine, or no obvious clinical attacks at all.

Continuous spike and wave complexes in sleep—
electrical status epilepticus in sleep (ESES)

This condition[148] refers to patients without paroxysms in the waking (or REM) state, but with nearly continuous, irregular, generalized spike and wave complexes at 1 to 2/sec. in slow wave sleep (see Fig. 6.31). The onset varies between 8 months to 12 years with a mean of 5 years. Either partial

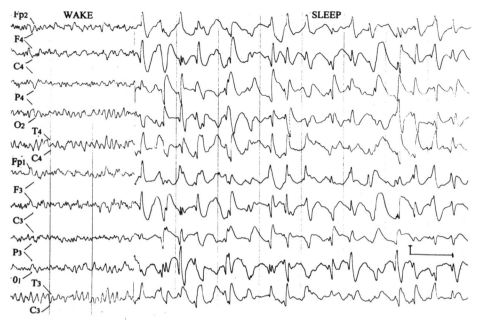

FIGURE 6.31   Electrical Status Epilepticus in Sleep (ESES). On the left note the wake record without epileptiform activity, but on the right during sleep nearly continuous irregular generalized spike and wave complexes are seen at 1.5–2/sec.

or generalized seizures may precede by 1 to 2 years this ESES, which is associated with a severe decrease in neurophysiological functions, including an absence of new learning. With appropriate anticonvulsant medication, especially benzodiazepines such as Clobazam (available in Europe and Canada), the pattern usually disappears by the teens. Because of the slow frequency and great abundance of these complexes, the Lennox-Gastaut Syndrome may be suspected, but patients with ESES are usually older and have no tonic attacks but more spike and wave complexes without polyspikes and without longer runs of polyspikes in the sleep record. One interesting aspect of this disorder is the relatively few cases in North America compared with the larger number reported in Europe.

Temporal sharp waves

Posterior Temporal (see Fig. 6.32)   Since this focus is close to and often associated with the occipital area, the age distribution is similar, usually with an onset of 5 to 8 years of age. The characteristics of the patients[149] are somewhat different from those with an occipital spike in that *clinical seizures* are more common and appear in almost three-quarters of the patients. Occasionally these children (8% of them) may have a focal motor seizure, as an indication that within that region, both laterally and mesially, motor responses are obtainable from stimulation. The most common type of seizure in this group is, however, a generalized tonic-clonic attack, and

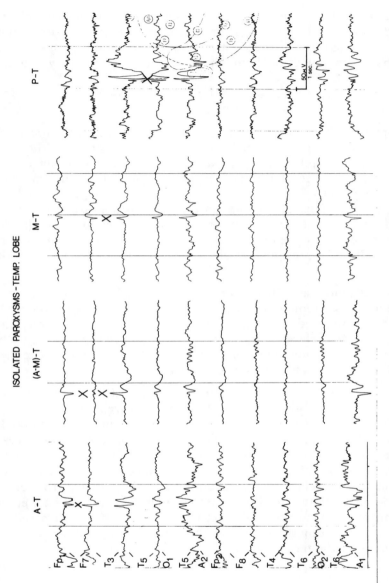

FIGURE 6.32   Single sharp wave discharges on the (four) temporal areas. Note the reversal on the (1) anterior (2) anterior-mid (equipotential), (3) mid, and (4) posterior temporal areas.

psychomotor spells are very uncommon (<2%). Neurovegetative phenomena in the form of headaches, dizzy spells, and blackouts are found in slightly over one-third of these patients and behavioral or psychological symptoms in one-fourth of them; the exact nature of these symptoms is, however, unclear.

Tegretol or Dilantin is often helpful in these patients and also in the other patients with temporal foci listed below.

Mid-temporal The mid-temporal focus is also seen in preadolescent children, but usually slightly older (6 to 10 years at onset) than those with posterior temporal spikes. These patients[149] often (56%) have *seizures*, but with a lower incidence than the other temporal foci listed in this section; however, they lead in incidence of *neurovegetative symptoms* (40%). Behavioral or psychological complaints are seen in approximately 18% of this group. Other distinctive features are the frequent presence (55%) of intermixed slow wave abnormalities, possibly related to a relatively high incidence (37%) of a presumed etiology (head injury) that is found in these patients.

Anterior-mid temporal This focus is equipotential between the anterior $(F_{7,8})$ and mid $(T_{3,4})$ temporal areas and clinically falls between the profiles of the anterior and mid-temporal groups.[149] Thus, *seizures* are noted in approximately 70% of these patients and *neurovegetative symptoms* in 39%. Psychological symptoms, however, are the least common of all temporal lobe discharges, with an incidence of only 12%.

Anterior temporal This focus is distinctive in that it is associated with the *highest incidence* (82%) *of seizures* (both of the psychomotor or complex partial and generalized tonic-clonic type) of any kind of temporal lobe discharge.[149] Since the incidence of clear clinical seizures and neurovegetative symptoms seems to be inversely related,[149] this focus is associated with the lowest incidence (25%) of the latter kinds of complaints. Psychological or behavioral symptoms are not uncommon (21%), although the relationship of these complaints to the seizure disorder continues to be a point of great controversy. One other distinctive feature is that intermixed slow waves are more commonly seen with the anterior temporal focus than any other focus from the temporal lobe.

Frontal sharp waves—frontal lobe epilepsy

These discharges (see Fig. 6.33) are more often seen in adults than children and the kinds of seizures in these patients can be in many different forms. Many (60%) have generalized tonic-clonic attacks and some (one-third) have tonic posturing, at times with gestural (repetitive movements) or vocal automatisms that can appear aggressive. Because of this type of clinical manifestation, these attacks are often mistaken for psychogenic or pseudoseizures. In addition, forced thinking or neurovegetative symptoms like

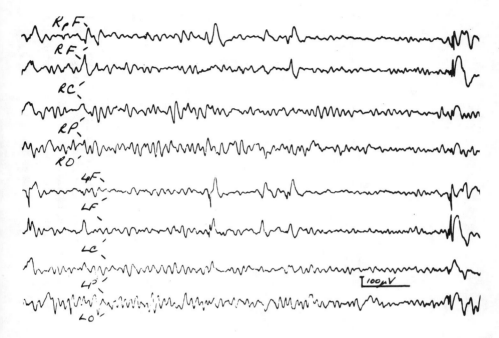

FIGURE 6.33   Frontal sharp waves. Note on Channels 1 and 2 on the right frontal area and Channels 5 and 6 on the left frontal area the sharp waves in a patient with frontal lobe epilepsy.

flushing can be a manifestation. Another clinical manifestation can be the contralateral movement of the head and eyes, at times with the arm raised as if the patient is looking at that arm. Jacksonian seizures with a march from a distal part, like the thumb, to more proximal parts, up the arm to the shoulder, are usually part of frontal lobe epilepsy.

Midline spikes—simple partial motor seizures

These spikes[150] can appear in children or adults (mean age, 23 years) and often (69%) are associated with focal motor seizures that maintain awareness and therefore are called *simple* partial attacks. A prominent negative phase is seen in about one-half, only a positive phase in some (13%), and both phases in about one-third.

Periodic lateralized epileptiform discharges (PLEDS)[151] (see Fig. 6.34)

This pattern has been called other names, such as Periodically Recurring Focal Discharges,[152] and refers to a *unilateral focus that continually and periodically fires throughout the entire tracing, usually at the frequency of 1 to 2/sec.* Commonly, the focus is posterior in location, especially on the

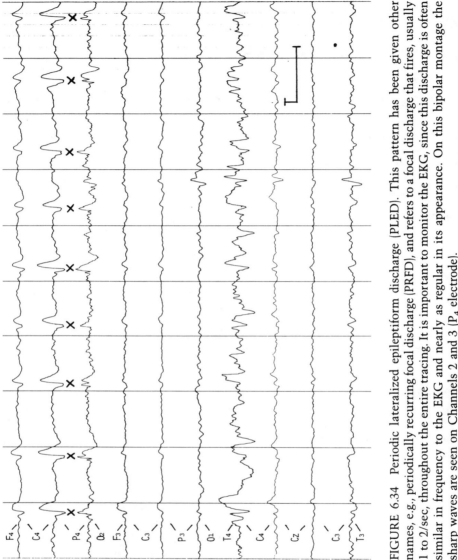

FIGURE 6.34 Periodic lateralized epileptiform discharge (PLED). This pattern has been given other names, e.g., periodically recurring focal discharge (PRFD), and refers to a focal discharge that fires, usually 1 to 2/sec, throughout the entire tracing. It is important to monitor the EKG, since this discharge is often similar in frequency to the EKG and nearly as regular in its appearance. On this bipolar montage the sharp waves are seen on Channels 2 and 3 (P₄ electrode).

parietal areas, but can be located in any given region. The pattern, of course, represents an extremely active focus, firing with single discharges at the maximum rate that such foci can discharge, viz., at 1 to 2/sec. At times, an *epilepsia partialis continua* is associated with the discharge, referring to the continually recurring jerking movement of certain muscle groups tied to the EEG discharge. The etiology of these PLEDS is most often *cerebrovascular* (often emboli), but a space-occupying lesion (especially *metastases*) is the second most common cause of these foci.[151,152] Clinical seizures are found in the majority of these patients (85%) and often can be predicted by the presence of fast rhythms between the discharges called "PLEDS PLUS."[153] The repetitive rate of the PLEDS contributes to the *degree* of disorientation or confusion of the patient. As the patient improves on drugs such as Dilantin or Tegretol and the discharge slows down, the patient will usually improve in degree of alertness and orientation.

Bilateral periodic sharp waves at 1 sec—
Jakob-Creutzfeldt disease (JCD)

These complexes (see Fig. 6.35) develop late in this disease and may resemble bilateral spike and wave complexes of a corticoreticular seizure disorder, but without a clear wave component because this latter projection system is probably involved. Differences are that in JCD the complexes are often nearly continuous, rather than in bursts, with a poorly developed wave, a more prominent spike component, maximal on the frontal areas, on a near nonexistent background rhythm. By 10 to 12 weeks after the initial onset of symptoms of JCD, this pattern will be present in the great majority of patients. Demented patients without this pattern whose symptoms have started more than 10 to 12 weeks before likely do not have JCD. This pattern usually appears at the time when myoclonic jerks are also seen.[154]

Repetitive irregular spike and wave complexes
with a depressed background—cerebral anoxia

These irregular complexes[155] are seen on the flat background and are like a suppression burst pattern (see Fig. 5.11) but with the bursts usually less than 1 second in duration. The pattern usually is seen in patients who have suffered significant cerebral anoxia, often from a cardiopulmonary arrest. Brief myoclonic jerks are often noted in these patients who are in a deeply comatose state. Their prognosis is so extremely poor that any kind of recovery is rare.

Controversial Sharp Waves or Spikes

Positive spikes at 6 to 7 and 14/sec (see Fig. 6.36)

Many electroencephalographers would claim that this pattern should not be discussed as a controversial waveform, since it is clearly normal.[156] On the other hand, others will claim (some only privately) that positive spikes are

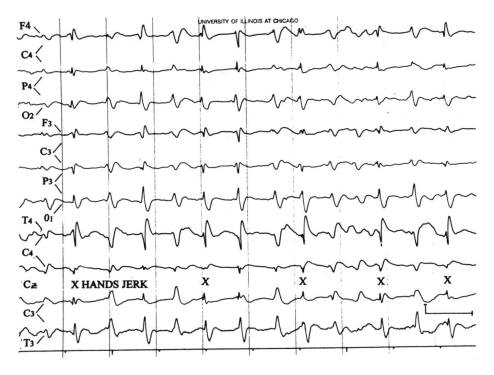

FIGURE 6.35   Bilateral periodic sharp waves at 1/sec, as seen in Jakob-Creutzfeldt Disease. Note the sharp waves that are synchronous between the two sides, usually maximal on the frontocentral areas at 1/sec and associated often with the myoclonic jerks of the hands.

likely significant.[94] Since the original description by Gibbs and Gibbs in 1951,[157] no pattern has aroused more intensive controversy than this one. Reviews published in 1963 (Henry)[158] and 1965 (Hughes)[159] emphasized as *possible* correlates *neurovegetative* symptoms, such as headaches, dizzy spells, blackouts, paroxysmal abdominal pains, and also *behavior disorders*, especially impulsive, acting-out behavior. Since that time scores of other papers have been published, some with positive findings and others with negative conclusions. One study[160] illustrates how easily negative conclusions can be drawn from a study on positive spikes on the one hand but, on the other hand, how positive correlations can appear after more careful study of the same patients. After careful clinical screening of hundreds of children to obtain a "normal" group, any EEG pattern found in this group could be viewed as "normal." In this group about 16% showed positive spikes, a finding that could be regarded as clinically insignificant. However, these same patients were then studied more carefully by pediatric psychiatrists who found significant relationships between the presence of these

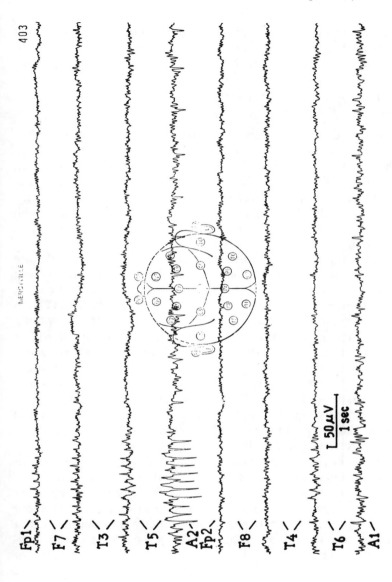

FIGURE 6.36 Positive spikes at 6 to 7 and 14/sec. This burst shows the slow 6 to 7/sec form, higher in amplitude and longer in duration than usual. The spikes are seen best on Channel 4 (referential linkage from the left posterior temporal area to the opposite ear) and show their positivity on this linkage by a downward direction. Note the upward deflections on Channels 1 through 3, indicating that each of those channels is reflecting a negative to positive polarity relationship.

positive spikes and various neurovegetative and behavioral disorders. This pattern, however, is not related to clinical seizures and is called a normal variant by many electroencephalographers.

Rhythmic mid-temporal discharges (RMTD) or psychomotor variant (PMV) (see Fig. 6.37)

This pattern was called *psychomotor variant* by Gibbs and Gibbs in 1952.[94] The same pattern was renamed *rhythmic mid-temporal discharges* by Lipman and Hughes in 1969[161] to avoid the use of clinical terms to describe an electrographic event, following the dictum of the International Federation for EEG and Clinical Neurophysiology to separate clinical and EEG terminology. The same initials, RMTD, have been maintained by others who have changed the *D* (for *Discharge*) to stand for activity in *Drowsiness*. The same group has maintained that this pattern is only a normal variant and therefore the term *Discharge*, implying abnormality, must be changed. One major problem with the *D* for *Drowsiness* is that, like all other sharp wave discharges, they appear best in *most* patients in the drowsy or light sleep stage, but at times do clearly appear in a wake state. Thus, the RMTD can hardly be a normal *drowsy* pattern if it can be clearly seen in the waking state of some patients. This waveform is also controversial, primarily for the same reason that all patterns in this section are—viz., they *do not highly correlate with seizures.* The incidence of seizures, either psychomotor or generalized tonic-clonic in form, was 33% according to Gibbs and Gibbs,[81] 36% (Lipman and Hughes),[161] and 27% (Hughes).[149] *Neurovegetative* symptoms, especially headaches, were more common at 60 to 63% and *psychological* complaints were noted in 47% (Lipman and Hughes) or 33% (Hughes). In the latter study psychological symptoms were more common in this group than in any of the seven other groups with some type of temporal lobe discharge. One other distinctive feature is that head injury (concussion) more often occurred in these patients (24%) than with any other type of temporal discharge. One fascinating feature is that many of these patients show *bizarre behavior* that appears superficially as a manifestation of a (psychological) behavior disorder, but also may have aspects that suggest complex partial seizures. Examples from the author's own patients include setting off fire alarms without any stimulus or provocation or violently striking an animal by a patient who is otherwise intact psychologically. This interesting pattern may represent a bridge between neurology and psychiatry, especially since patients with the RMTD pattern often show somatization of complaints and abnormal MMPIs.[162,163]

Hughes and Cayaffa[164] found that patients with RMTD tended either to *fail to respond or to increase their latency of responding to an external stimulus* when that stimulus was presented *during a burst of RMTD.* These data supported the possibility that this pattern may really be an ictal phenomenon but with only subtle clinical manifestations.

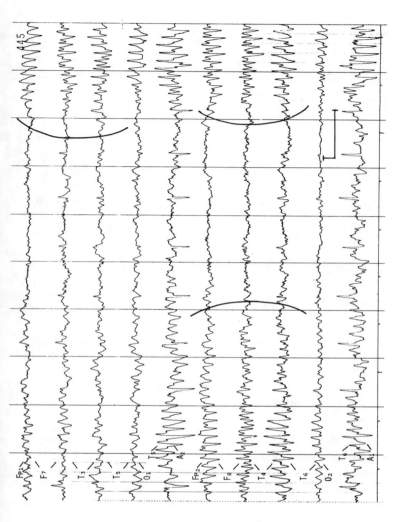

FIGURE 6.37 Rhythmic–mid-temporal discharges (RMTD)—known as *psychomotor variant*. The phase reversal between Channels 2 and 3 on the left and between Channels 7 and 8 on the right indicates that the mid-temporal regions (T3,4) are maximally involved with these discharges, which usually appear at 5–6/sec with a harmonic of 10–12/sec, seen as faster activity intermixed with the slower form. Usually both the left and right temporal areas show these bursts in any given record as noted here, on the right and later on the left, quickly transmitted to the right.

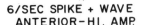

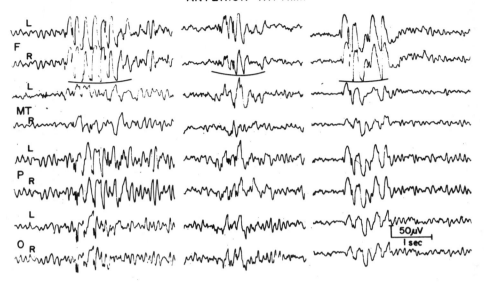

FIGURE 6.38   The 6/sec spike and wave complex (WHAM form). Note the complexes in the *waking* record, *high* in amplitude and *anterior* in location, seen in this *male* patient with clinical seizures.

The 6/sec spike and wave complex
(see Figs. 6.38 and 6.39)

This pattern is difficult to recognize, often very low in amplitude and rare in appearance, contributing to its controversial nature. Confusion in the literature likely arises because there are really *two types* of 6/sec spike and wave complexes.[165] Some authors studied more of one form, because of their own distinctive patient population, while other investigators studied the other form, leading to significant differences and confusion in the literature. From a large number (839) of these patients collected over decades and present in the extensive files of the University of Illinois Medical Center, the author has found the two forms, WHAM and FOLD, representing two ends of a continuum, along which any one patient may be found. WHAM is an acronym referring to patients with this pattern found in *Waking* record, *High* in amplitude, *Anterior* in location, and found more in *Males*. The WHAM form is found mainly in patients with *seizures*. The FOLD form appears mainly in *Females*, maximal on the *Occipital* areas, *Low* in amplitude, and in the *Drowsy* state. This form appears in patients with *neurovegetative* and *psychological* complaints, and is the controversial form because of the latter types of symptoms. For nearly four decades the author has searched for a 6/sec spike and wave complex with a sufficiently long duration that the responsiveness of the patient could be tested. Since there are many similar-

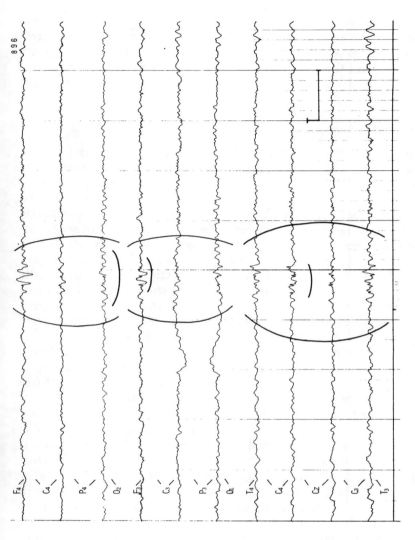

FIGURE 6.39   The 6/sec spike and wave complex, (FOLD form) Note the bilateral symmetry of this low amplitude complex, appearing well on Channels 1 (right frontal) and 4 (left frontal), and also seen similarly on Channels 9 and 10 on the left as well as 7 and 8 on the right. This example is the low amplitude form usually associated with neurovegetative and psychological complaints, more commonly seen than the high amplitude form, usually associated with convulsions.

ities between the 6/sec and 3/sec forms, often seen together in the same patient, the appropriate test was to see if there was a change in responsiveness during the 6/sec form. In one patient with the longest complexes yet seen, the data[166] were clear that, like the 3/sec form, a significantly long latency of response appeared during the duration of the 6/sec spike and wave complex.

Small sharp spikes (SSS) (see Fig. 6.40)

This pattern was described by Gibbs and Gibbs,[81] who considered it "an epileptic abnormality," but Reiher and Klass[167] viewed it as a "pattern of doubtful significance" and White and colleagues[168] renamed the waveform "benign epileptiform transients of sleep" (BETS) to emphasize that it is essentially normal. The same three kinds of symptoms have been previously reported for the SSS, as have been discussed for the other controversial patterns, namely seizures, neurovegetative and psychological complaints.

The incidence of *seizures* has varied from 72% (Gibbses)[81] to 67% (Koshino and Niedermeyer)[169] and to 42% in a recent study of 300 cases by the present reviewer.[149] One conclusion in this latter study was that this pattern was associated with only a *moderate seizure tendency*. In this same study *neurovegetative* symptoms were also *moderate* in incidence, viz., 48%, but psychological complaints appeared in only 16%.

Recent data have made more clear why some investigators have found this waveform associated with seizures and others have not. At least two important variables determine seizure incidence. First is age with a linear inverse relationship between age and the incidence with definite clinical seizures.[170] Teenagers with SSS had an 80% incidence of seizures and octogenarians had a 0% incidence, with a relatively straight line between these two extreme age groups. The age and seizure data of Koshino and Niedermeyer were plotted on the latter curve and demonstrated this same clear relationship with age. No data on age were published with the study by White et al. The second variable is the number of SSS.[171] Patients with more than 2/min usually had seizures and those with less than 1/min did not. Thus, the variable of how active the SSS were proved important, as one would expect from the common sense or intuitive point of view. Another important point is that, like all other phenomena in our world, discharges do not conveniently fall into two groups of typical spikes and small sharp spikes. There is every imaginable gradation between the two groups and SSS should be designated only when they fit the original description of Gibbs and Gibbs who named them.

Wicket temporal spikes (see Fig. 6.41)

This pattern was first described by Reiher and Lebel[172] and refers to temporal spikes that may appear as single isolated events, but also are seen in *bursts*, usually at theta frequencies, especially 5 to 7.5/sec. The latter

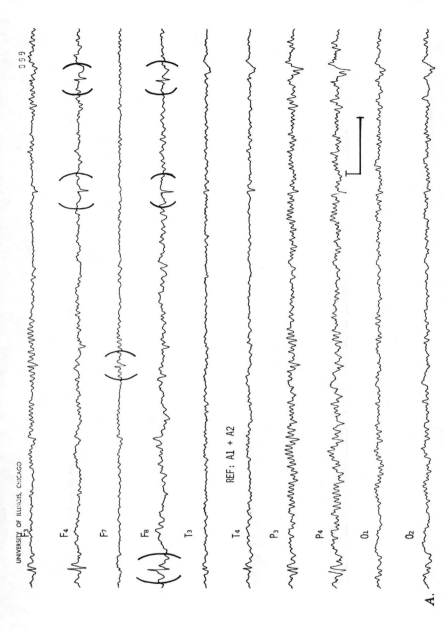

FIGURE 6.40 *A.* Small sharp spikes. On the referential recording (to both ears) note the sharp discharges on the left and right sides, maximal on the frontal or anterior temporal areas. *B.* On a bipolar recording.

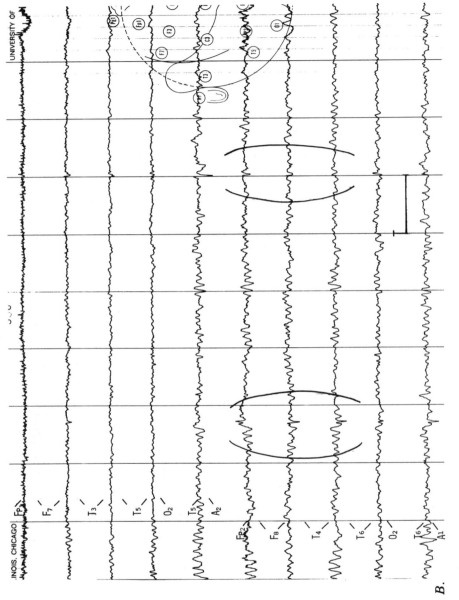

B.

FIGURE 6.40 *(continued)*

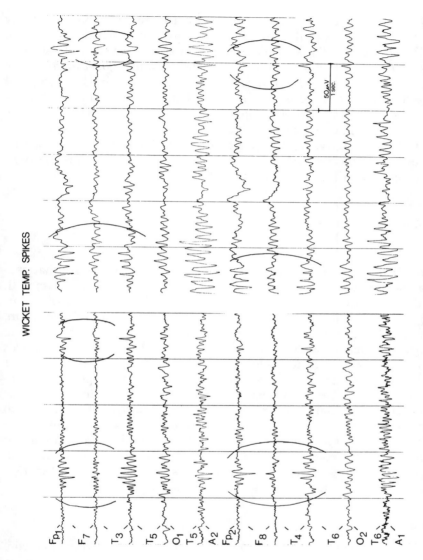

FIGURE 6.41 Wicket temporal sharp waves. Note that these sharp waves occur singly and also in a burst, often at the theta frequency of 5 to 7.5/sec.

authors concluded that this pattern did not correlate with epilepsy or any other symptom complex, although 80% did have nonepileptic symptoms, especially syncope (33%), headaches, and vertigo. In a study published by the present reviewer,[149] the wicket pattern showed the *highest incidence of neurovegetative symptoms* (70%) of all eight different kinds of temporal lobe discharge. This pattern also had the highest incidence in *females* (62%), often with some type of etiology (40%), especially head injury (22%). The incidence of seizures was 38%, suggesting a *moderate epileptogenic potential*. Other distinctive features were that wicket temporal spikes, with a *peak age around the seventh decade,* never were found only on the right side and were either left-sided or bilateral.

Other Specific Patterns

Triphasic Waves

The name *triphasic*[173] is the most popular name for this waveform that usually is associated with *liver* disorders affecting the brain, but patients with other diffuse disorders, especially *uremia,*[174] may also show the same pattern (Fig. 6.42). Although "triphasic" is the most commonly used term, other terms that are more descriptive are "blunt spike and wave"[175] and "pseudoparoxysmal spike and wave,"[176] indicating that the bursts of waves have a spikelike configuration before each wave, but without the sharpness of the classical 3/sec spike and wave complexes of absence ("petit mal") epilepsy. The term *triphasic* is imperfect since it is not immediately obvious to most electroencephalographers what the three phases of this waveform are, consisting otherwise of a blunted spike and a slow wave complex. The waveform is seen in *some* patients in impending or frank hepatic coma, but its absence does not rule out hepatic disease. Triphasic waves are not usually seen in patients who are awake, nor in those in deep coma, but instead in patients in a just-arousable stage of semicoma.

EEG in Subacute Sclerosing Panencephalitis (SSPE)

The SSPE pattern is nearly pathognomonic of this serious disorder and consists of *short bursts of irregular, bilateral sharp and slow wave complexes, appearing periodically, usually every 5 to 6 seconds*[177] (Fig. 6.43). Their periodicity has been studied by many investigators,[177] but to date they do not seem to be associated with any particular physiological variable.

Extreme Spindles[81]

This term refers to sleep patterns (Fig. 6.44) that are much more exaggerated than the common spindle (sigma) activity which usually has a duration up to 4 seconds in normals. Extreme spindles have a relatively *high amplitude*

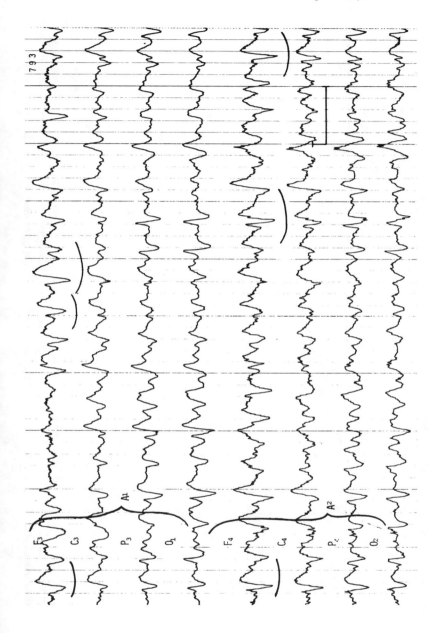

FIGURE 6.42 Triphasic waves. This pattern, seen especially in hepatic (and renal) coma, is like a blunted spike and wave complex, exemplified by the portions underlined. Usually the pattern is diffuse, but maximal on the frontal areas and usually is seen in bursts.

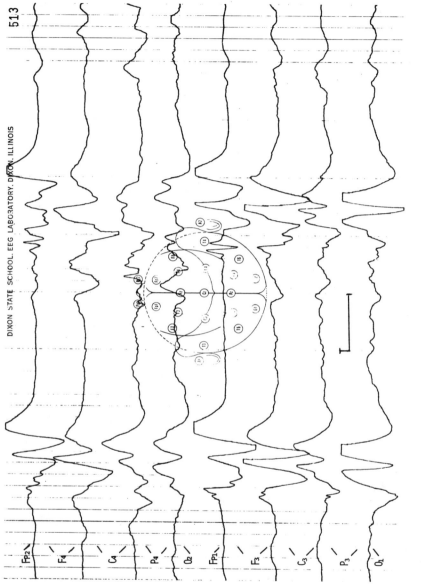

FIGURE 6.43   Subacute sclerosing panencephalitis (SSPE). This distinctive pattern consists of short bursts of irregular sharp and slow wave complexes, appearing periodically, often every 5 to 6 seconds in duration throughout the entire tracing, against a depressed background rhythm. (See next page for continuation.)

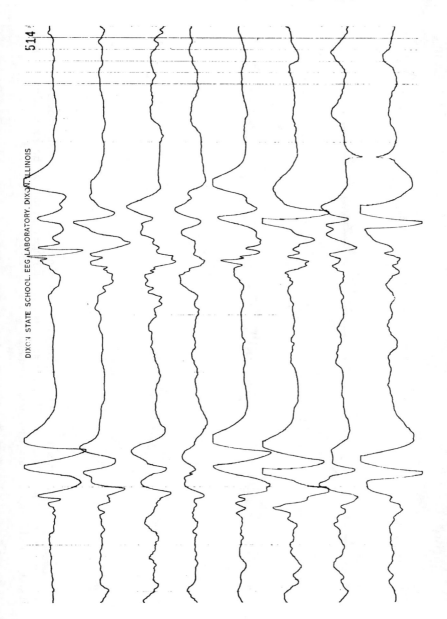

FIGURE 6.43 *(continued)*

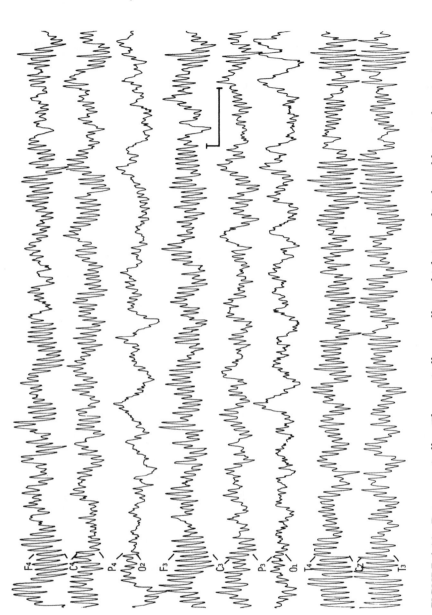

FIGURE 6.44   Extreme spindles. These spindles usually are high in amplitude and long in duration, as seen here, lasting more than 10 seconds. They appear diffuse, but often are maximal on the frontal (Channel 1 and 4) and central vertex regions (Channels 7 and 8).

and sometimes a slower frequency than the normal spindle, but a simple rule that will easily identify the pattern is that spindles lasting for *longer* than one EEG page (longer than 10 seconds) usually are extreme spindles. They should not be so identified if the patient is taking some type of benzodiazepine medication (Librium, Valium, etc.) or barbiturate, since the EEG of these patients will also show longer lasting spindles of similar frequency—about 14/sec.[178] Extreme spindles are related to *mental subnormality;*[56] their presence should not be used to *predict* this clinical condition, but only to support or confirm a known mental retardation in the form of an electroclinical correlation.

Mitten Pattern (See Fig. 6.45)

This pattern, according to certain authors,[81] has been divided into the A and B forms, depending on whether the "thumb" of the mitten is ⅛ to ⅑ of a second in duration, often associated with Parkinsonism, or ⅒ to 1/12/sec, associated with psychoses. If the "thumb" is even slower, at ⅙ to 1/7/sec, the association is with disorders involving deep (thalamic) structures. The mitten pattern, however, is *clearly* controversial and is rarely ever mentioned in present day EEG interpretations.

Frontal Arousal Rhythm (FAR)[179]

This pattern is extremely rare (see Fig. 6.46), but when it does occur is seen in children with *seizures and/or learning disabilities.*

Summary of Abnormal EEG Patterns and Associated Clinical Conditions

The reader is reminded that the EEG findings and the associated clinical conditions are based on *statistical relationships* and some are obviously stronger than others. Therefore, the following represent in *no* way electroclinical correlations that are 100% predictable, but instead are relationships that are anticipated or expected and should at least be carefully considered by the clinician.

Depression of Normal Rhythms or Slow Waves

There are nonspecific findings that can reflect any organic neuronal condition, involving a focal area, all of one hemisphere or both hemispheres.

1. Diffuse slow—especially metabolic, toxic, infectious etiologies.
    (a) If symmetrical—projected disturbance from near-midline, subcortical regions.

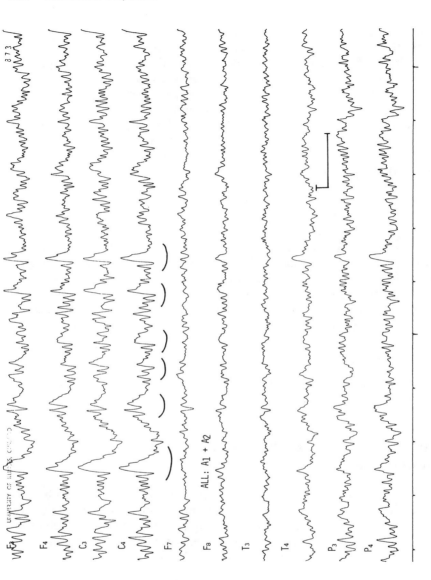

FIGURE 6.45   Mitten pattern. This pattern looks like a mitten with a short "thumb" followed by wider slow waves, exemplified by the underlined portions on Channels 3 and 4, and often appear in bursts.

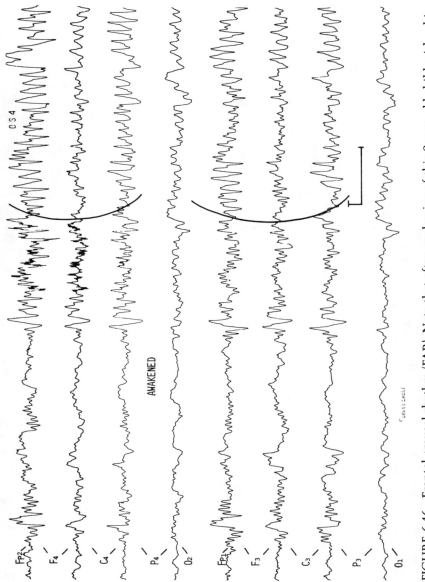

FIGURE 6.46   Frontal arousal rhythm (FAR). Note that after awakening of this 9-year-old child with a history of generalized seizures, sharp waves are seen bifrontally in a long burst at 5/sec.

    (b) Decreased background frequency—any diffuse disturbance, including senility, hypothyroidism.

2. Focal slow—if very slow, consider space-occupying lesion.

    (a) Frontal

        (i)   FIRDA—anterior brain stem disturbance, including midline tumors, metabolic, infectious, degenerative disorders.

        (ii) Abnormal theta—same as FIRDA but less severe.

        (iii) Unilateral—with temporal-vascular involving the ipsilateral carotid artery (CVA).

    (b) Temporal—most common EEG finding, more often on left side, often in senility, anoxic conditions, head injury.

    (c) Parietal—consider space-occupying lesion, especially in adults.

    (d) Occipital—nonspecific in children, at times in learning disabilities, if very slow-posterior fossa tumor. In adults with temporal slowing—vertebral-basilar insufficiency.

Sharp Paroxysmal Activity

Neonatal

1. Negative sharp waves or spikes—seizures.
2. Positive central or temporal sharp waves—intraventricular hemorrhage, periventricular leukomalacia, infarcts, only at times with seizures.
3. Repetitive spikes—clonic seizures.
4. Slow delta discharges—tonic seizures.
5. Theta pointu alternant—5th day seizures.

Postnatal

1. Suppression burst—early infantile epileptic encephalopathy (EIEE) or neonatal myoclonic encephalopathy.
2. Hypsarrhythmia—infantile spasms.
3. Slow (1 to 2/sec) spike and wave—Lennox-Gastaut Syndrome (tonic seizures).
4. 3/sec spike and wave complexes—absence (multiple spike: generalized tonic-clonic seizure).
    (a) Irregular—atonic, myoclonic attacks.
5. Occipital sharp waves—benign occipital epilepsy, retrolental fibroplasia (rare), visual perceptual disorders.
6. Centrotemporal sharp waves—benign epilepsy of childhood.
7. Parietal sharp waves—versive or sensory seizures.
8. Prefrontal sharp waves—neurovegetative seizures.
9. Bioccipital spike and wave complexes—partial and generalized seizures (and migraine).
10. Electrical Status Epilepticus of Sleep (ESES)—no new learning.

11. Frontal sharp waves—Jacksonian or versive seizures or repetitive movements.
12. Midline sharp waves—simple partial seizures.
13. Temporal sharp waves.
    (a) Posterior—neurovegetative symptoms and seizures.
    (b) Mid—neurovegetative symptoms and seizures.
    (c) Anterior—seizures (complex partial and generalized tonic-clonic).
14. Periodic lateralized epileptiform discharges (PLED)—epilepsia partialis continua—cerebrovascular (emboli) and also (metastatic) tumors.
15. Bilateral periodic sharp waves at 1/sec—Jakob-Creutzfeldt Disease.
16. Repetitive irregular spike and wavelike complexes with a depressed background—cerebral anoxia.
17. Controversial patterns.
    (a) 6 to 7 and 14/sec positive spikes—adolescents with neurovegetative and behavior disorders (?) or normal variant.
    (b) Rhythmic mid-temporal discharges (RMTD)—(psychomotor variant)—bizarre behavior, subtle ictal pattern?
    (c) 6/sec spike and wave—WHAM form: seizures; FOLD form: neurovegetative and psychological symptoms.
    (d) Small sharp spikes (SSS)—also called (benign) epileptiform transients of sleep (BETS).
    (e) Wicket temporal spikes—older patients with syncope.
18. Other periodic or repetitive patterns.
    (a) Triphasic—hepatic (renal) coma.
    (b) Periodic burst (every 4 to 8 seconds)—subacute sclerosing panencephalitis (SSPE).
        (i) Periodic temporal sharp waves—herpes simplex encephalitis.
    (c) Extreme spindles: mental subnormality.
    (d) Mitten pattern—controversial—Parkinsonism (?), psychosis (?).
    (e) Frontal arousal rhythm (FAR)—learning disorders or seizures (children).

Summary of Abnormal Clinical Conditions and Associated EEG Patterns

Metabolic, Infectious, Toxic Etiologies

These are diffuse slow waves, decreased frequency of background rhythm, FIRDA

1. Hepatic (renal) coma—triphasic waves.
2. Subacute sclerosing panencephalitis (SSPE)—periodic bursts every 4 to 6 seconds.
3. Repetitive discharge, such as a PLED on the temporal lobe—herpes simplex encephalitis.

Vascular

1. CVA or TIA.
    (a) Carotid—frontal and temporal slow waves, more often on the left.
    (b) Vertebrobasilar—temporal and occipital slow waves.
        (i) Also FIRDA, desynchronized low amplitude record.
2. Hemorrhage.
    (a) Often sharp waves or spikes, in addition to slow waves.
3. Emboli.
    (a) Often parietal in location, at times periodic lateralized epileptiform discharges (PLEDs).
4. Subdural hematoma.
    (a) Slow waves, usually appearing after depression of normal rhythms.

Space-Occupying Lesion

1. Abscess—highly localized, very abnormal slow waves (over area with abscess).
2. Tumor.
    (a) Depth of lesion.
        (i) Deep—more rhythmical—at times theta frequencies.
        (ii) Superficial—more irregular, delta waves, suppression of normal background rhythm, consider especially if EEG "worse" than clinical picture. Polymorphic delta (PMD) waves.
    (b) Midline—bilaterally synchronous slow waves maximal frontal (anterior brainstem) or occipital (posterior brainstem).
        (i) Posterior fossa (children).
            1. Irregular shifting delta waves (occipital).
            2. Regular delta waves (occipital).
            3. Also frontal slowing.
            4. Also bilateral parasagittal slowing.
    (c) Rate of growth.
        (i) Slow—sharp waves with slow waves.
        (ii) Fast—very slow waves only.

Senility

Decreased frequency of background rhythm, temporal slow waves, especially on the left side. Later diffuse delta rhythms maximal on the frontal areas.

Learning or Mental Disabilities

1. Frontal arousal rhythm (FAR)—rare.
2. Occipital slow waves.
3. Extreme spindles (mental subnormality—retardation).

Seizures

Neonatal

1. Intraventricular hemorrhage, leukomalacia, infarcts—positive central or temporal sharp waves.
2. Seizures—negative sharp waves.
3. "Epileptic" seizures—EEG ictal rhythms.
4. "Non-epileptic" seizures—no EEG ictal rhythms.

Postnatal

1. 5th day seizures—theta pointu alternant.
2. Early infantile epileptic encephalopathy (EIEE) or neonatal myoclonic encephalopathy—suppression burst.
3. Infantile spasms—hypsarrhythmia.
4. Lennox-Gastaut Syndrome—1 to 2/sec spike and wave complexes (petit mal variant).
5. Absence attacks—regular 3/sec spike and wave complexes bilaterally synchronous. Also, generalized tonic-clonic seizures—multiple spikes.
6. Myoclonic, atonic seizures—irregular 3/sec spike and wave complexes.
7. Benign epilepsy of childhood—central sharp waves.
8. Benign occipital epilepsy—occipital sharp waves.
9. Versive or sensory seizures—parietal sharp waves.
10. Focal motor or Jacksonian seizures—frontocentral sharp waves.
11. Complex partial seizures—temporal lobe sharp waves, especially from the anterior temporal area.

CHAPTER 7

Topics of Special Interest

Recording in Intensive Care Units

Recording Clear Activity in Comatose Patients

Recording conditions in intensive care units are usually suboptimal, but a few points to keep in mind may solve most of the problems encountered there. If a comatose patient is moving spontaneously, has cephalic (head) reflexes, and is breathing, the question asked of the EEG will not usually be whether there is a possible brain death, but instead the extent and localization of the cerebral disturbance. Under the latter circumstances, standard montages will likely be sufficient. Of course, if time permits, a full set of electrodes can be applied and many different runs can be used, but usually this luxury of time does not exist while recording in intensive care units. As long as all of these electrodes have a *similar* impedance, the recording will likely be acceptable, since it is *different* impedances between two electrodes contributing to a given channel that represents the major artifact problem, rather than a relatively high impedance value for those same two electrodes.

After the electrodes are in place, a useful maneuver is to gather the leads together from the electrodes and loosely wrap a towel around those wires to make certain that none will be waving in the breeze to create movement artifacts. Another significant problem can be 60 cycle artifact, appearing especially from ineffective grounds, and, when seen, the source must be found to eliminate this interference. Remember that an electrical apparatus need only be plugged into the wall socket, without actually being turned to the "on" position to produce 60 cycle artifact. The first maneuver is to remove systematically plugs from the wall socket (with permission from the proper authorities) to determine the offending apparatus and, if found, the solution will be to keep that apparatus unplugged. If this machine must remain plugged into that socket, then a separate ground lead from the apparatus to a good grounding point (water faucet) sometimes solves the problem, which appears usually only on older machines. If an EKG monitor is being run with its own ground, then another ground applied by the EEG technician should *not* be used, since current could run between those two grounds in the form of "ground loops." Some new machines have isolated grounds to avoid this type of problem. Without any other ground the patient needs a ground electrode from the EEG technician; one exception would be the patient with a cardiac catheter, who should not be grounded unless a machine with an isolated ground is used. At times, 60 cycle artifact or other electrical disturbances can be eliminated by shortening all cables as much as possible (placing the cable not in rings but in a few figure 8s), especially the one to the wall socket from the EEG machine. Spatial orientation of the EEG machine in the room can occasionally be important, and changes in its position can make a difference in a very directional 60 cycle artifact. One important responsibility of the technician is to write down notes on the record on all of the many environmental disturbances that occur so the electroencephalographer may know the sources of these artifacts that appear in this special complex situation.

Recording Possible Electrocerebral Silence (ECS) in
Comatose Patients

The problems just outlined for recording from a patient with clear EEG activity in an intensive care unit may be multiplied in patients with no spontaneous respiration and therefore on a respirator, no movements, no cephalic reflexes, and therefore with possible brain death. In these instances the sensitivity of the EEG machine will be at its maximum, and every conceivable artifact can be recorded. Among the many montages that have been used under these circumstances the electroencephalographers associated with the NIH Collaborative Study on Cerebral Death agreed that one in particular was superior to all others. This one montage is in most instances the only one needed in those patients in whom the question is presence or absence of brain death. The run for an eight-channel machine is F_p2 to C4, C4 to O2, F_p1 to C3, C3 to O1, T4 to Cz, and Cz to T3 for the last six channels of EEG. For a 10-channel machine two other *linkages* that can be added are F8 to T6 and F7 to T5. The second channel should be EKG from two electrodes 3 inches apart over the left chest wall. The first channel of this montage is crucial since it will indicate the amount of artifact in the whole environment. This channel will be from two *noncephalic* leads, namely from two electrodes (3 inches apart) on the hand.

Any activity recorded from the hand electrodes will, of course, be artifact and not brain activity, and this artifact on Channel 1 can usually be expected to be just as prominent in all of the EEG channels. This first channel from the hand must be exactly at the same sensitivity as the EEG channels and the technicians' effort should be directed at reducing all the artifact of this channel to a very bare minimum (<2 mm). When the first channel is then clear, the other EEG channels will likely also be relatively free of artifact; an ECS, if existent, can then be usually designated. On the other hand, the artifact from the first channel from the hand may be more than 2 to 4 mm in amplitude (at the highest sensitivity setting of 1 μV/mm). Then an existing ECS may not be determined, since the same amount of artifact can be expected on the EEG, which needs to be less than 2 μV in amplitude for an ECS determination. Thus, continuous artifact of questionable origin greater than 2 μV, as shown by the (hand) noncephalic leads, will not usually permit an appreciation of ECS when it does exist, since an ECS determination requires activity under 2 μV.

The sensitivity on the EKG channel will be very much reduced, compared to the other channels, since the heart sends out such a greater potential than the brain, especially in comatose patients with little or no activity from the brain. Note that the montage involves skipping over one electrode in a chain and engages every other electrode in that chain. The reason for the widely spaced electrodes is to maximize the opportunity of recording any activity if it does exist. Widely spaced electrodes effectively increase the amplitude of the existing rhythm. Closely spaced electrodes, by looking at similar rhythms, record low amplitudes since it is the *difference* between the rhythms from each electrode that is recorded.

If the clinical picture suggests brain death as a reasonable possibility, then only the electrodes designated in this latter montage need be applied. The major effort of the technician is now to eliminate as much vibration (see Fig. 7.1 *A, B*) as possible, especially that produced by the bolus of air as it is delivered through the tracheostomy tube. Usually, the placing of supporting towels around this tube and carefully isolating it from the body will reduce the head vibration, which is also usually picked up by the EEG electrodes. Towels also should be used to reduce the movement of the head as the chest wall moves up and down during the artificial respiration. With all vibration at a minimum and with all unnecessary plugs pulled out of the wall sockets the recording can begin at standard sensitivity. The sensitivity is then moved up and up until clear activity is recorded or the maximum setting (usually 1 μV/mm) is reached. When maximum sensitivity is reached, usually more adjustments need to be made to further minimize various artifacts associated with the artificial respiration (see Fig. 7.1 *C*). The technician should indicate on the record the onset of each respiration and, if necessary, place two electrodes on some moving part of the respirator and use one channel for recording the respirator artifact. Another technique is to place two electrodes on the (other) hand, not used as a noncephalic lead, to be placed on the moving chest or abdomen; with each inspiration the movement artifact from the excursion of this hand on the chest wall will usually indicate respiration.

One rule in these recordings is important: if an artifact from some movements cannot be eliminated, then put an electrode on the moving part and record the artifact to see if it is contaminating the brain waves. Thus, if the artifact cannot be controlled, then record it so its presence and absence are evident. If the right cheek is jerking to produce an artifact in the EEG recording, an electrode, typically placed on the face (nose, chin) for

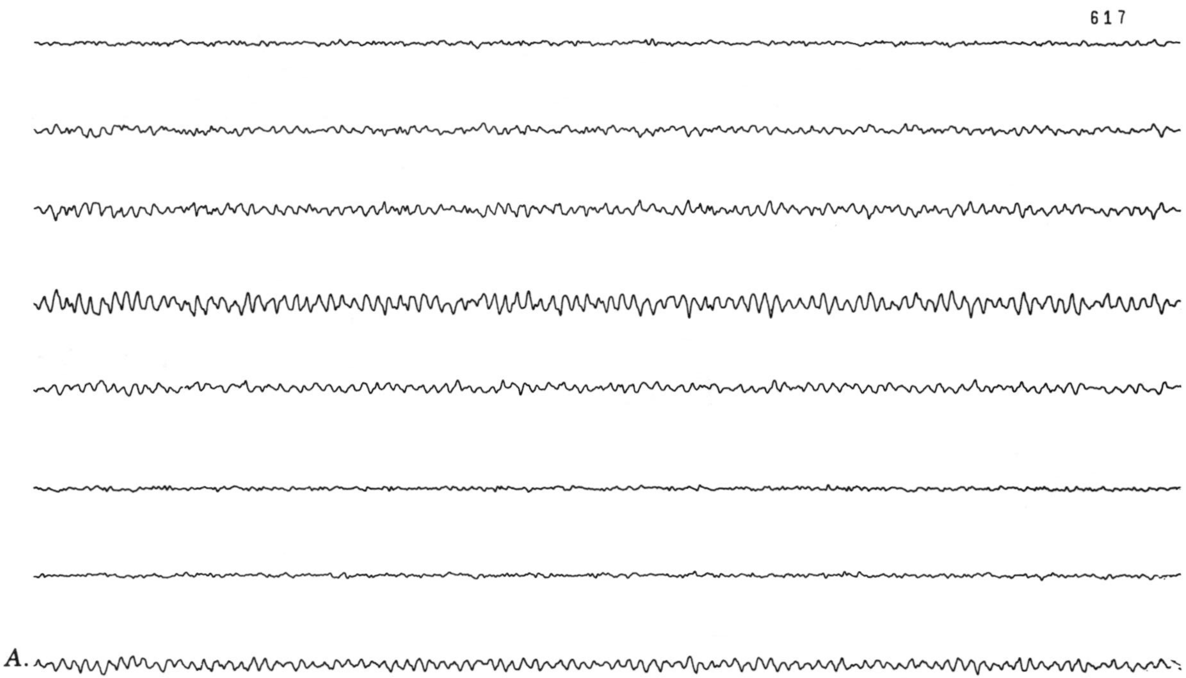

FIGURE 7.1   A. Vibration artifact and no brain waves. This remarkable record was obtained after a patient suddenly removed himself from all connections with the EEG machine. The rhythms, similar in appearance to normal alpha, likely are the result of vibration of the leads hanging in the air and underscore the importance of properly identifying vibration or tremor artifact. B. Tremor. Note the rhythmical 7/sec activity at very high gain settings appearing as brain activity. C. After the body tremor was minimized, note that nearly all of these 7/sec (artifactual) rhythms have disappeared. Underlined are remaining pulse artifacts, which are evident by checking the EKG on Channel 2.

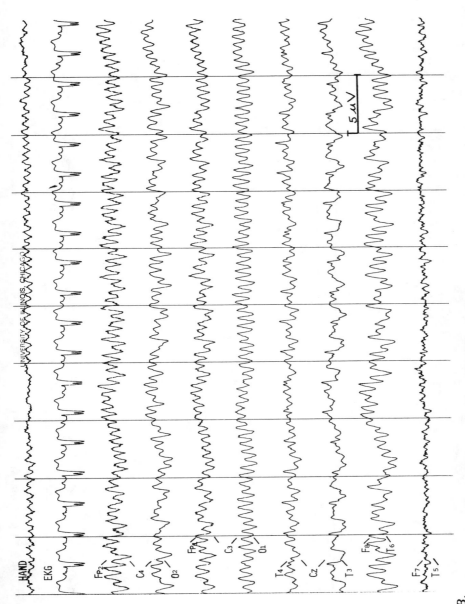

B. FIGURE 7.1 *(continued)*

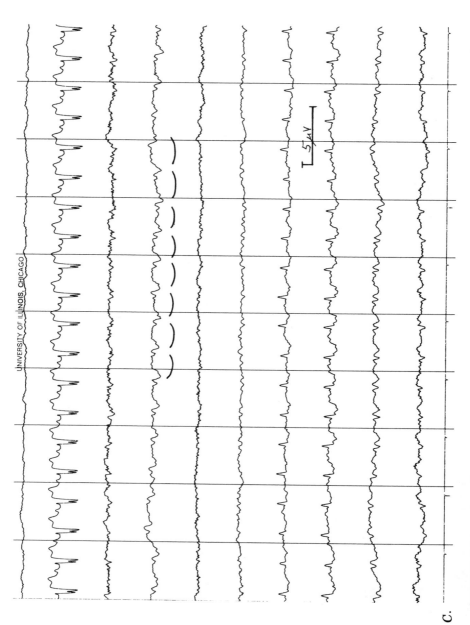

FIGURE 7.1 (*continued*)

monitoring most head movements, may not record this artifact properly. An electrode directly on the moving part, the cheek, will then be necessary.

Once an interpretable EEG can be obtained, then 30 minutes of actual recording time is necessary. At the very highest sensitivity settings used, it is important for the technicians to write on the record all of the many interferences that will influence the EEG. The eyes of the technicians should be fixed onto the record and they should constantly be correlating any changes seen on the record with changes in the environment of the patient, from the ringing of a telephone to a nurse walking by the bed. Thus, it is clear that satisfactory records in the intensive care unit will require the expertise of a highly qualified EEG technician. Novice technicians will need considerable training in this environment, but experienced technicians can learn to run excellent records in a relatively short time by close attention to the previous points and to solid principles behind good EEG technique. The problems in obtaining satisfactory records in intensive care units should *never* be considered so overwhelming that they provide an excuse for downgrading the usefulness of an EEG in coma or possible brain death.

Special problems can be encountered in the premature or neonatal intensive care unit. Since the heads of these patients are tiny, proper electrode placement is likely more crucial, and smaller amounts of electrode conducting paste may be required to avoid overlapping the paste from two areas and creating a bridge between them. Special care should be given to avoid bridging from the ground electrode to a nearby active scalp electrode, a situation that can create 60 cycle artifact. The resistance or impedance of the electrodes often needs to be especially low, since more electrical apparatus capable of producing artifacts usually surrounds these patients. To avoid movement of the wires from the electrodes, paper tape can be used to secure lightly the proximal portion of these wires to the head, bringing them together in the form of a cap.

If an IV is placed in a scalp vein, its position should be drawn on a head diagram and special attention should be given to any periodic patterns in the EEG as possible drip artifacts or to a depression of activity from a possible infiltration. Since high humidity or wetness in the area tends to exacerbate the technical problems in obtaining a satisfactory EEG, removal of wet diapers and replacing them with dry ones is important, as is replacing the damp cloths often found under oxygen hoods.

Since infants often show jitteriness that can cause artifacts, it is often advisable to wrap the baby loosely in a towel without grossly restricting the movements. This technique should not, of course, be used in infants with possible seizures, since their seizures may not then be viewed. In general, everything seems more concentrated in these neonatal intensive care units, so greater efficiency on the part of the EEG technician seems required. A good policy is for the technician to establish excellent rapport with the head nurse, getting ready for the EEG recording, and then asking her if nursing responsibilities can be carried out before the recording, which should then be run as much in a continuous manner as possible.

Common Problems in EEG Laboratories Requiring Discussion Between Technicians and Physician-Electroencephalographers

The following problems are discussed since experience shows them to be the most common sources of difficulty in EEG departments and most books do not deal with these matters. The physician-electroencephalographer should therefore discuss these practical problems with technicians to avoid the pitfalls so outlined.

Identification of the EEG Record

Make certain that the *identification of the EEG record* is with the *correct* name and also correct EEG requisition. Proper identification of each record is mainly the responsibility of the EEG technician. If the wrong name is placed on the record, its discovery may not be picked up by the electroencephalographer whose responsibilities are not oriented to pick up this kind of mistake. If the wrong requisition is placed with a given record, the report may be dictated, using the name on that requisition rather than the one on the face sheet of the EEG record. Fortunately, these mistakes do not occur often, but when they do they can be serious and very embarrassing.

History of the Patient

Provide (or add) history of the patient on the EEG requisition. Directors of EEG departments are forever writing memos to referring physicians, pleading for more (or any) clinical information on the patient scheduled for an EEG. At times, however, none will be available when the patient arrives for the recording. All technicians should learn to take a good history and to add to what is given on the EEG requisition. If the patient is not communicative, at least the technician should determine the major problem for which the patient was referred.

Sleep Medication

Give sleep medication (chloral hydrate) *only to alert patients* and not to a lethargic or drowsy patient. Usually, the technician has the responsibility of judging the need for medication for a sleep record. Although the EEG requisition may provide permission for the use of this medication, this permission does not mean that the drug should necessarily be given. If the patient believes that natural sleep can be obtained, of course, it should be attempted. Good advice to technicians who administer medication is that they can always give more, but they cannot take out what has already been given. Approximately 25 to 30 minutes should be given to evaluate the effect of a given oral dose before giving any more of the medication.

Calibration

Make certain that *all channels are appropriately recording* during machine calibration or patient calibration. EEG technicians are engaged in two types of tasks, one highly routine and the other highly cognitive. On the one hand, they measure each head the same way on each patient, place the electrodes on the scalp the same way each time, provide the same kind of information on each record and on each montage, etc. On the other hand, they must change gears from routinized tasks to ones that require careful observation of the EEG record followed by action based on the information obtained. Some technicians allow the routine part of their professional life to overlap the part that should be cognitive, requiring concentration and thought. Therefore, calibration of the machine becomes too routine, and, as such, no careful inspection may be made of this part of the record. At the time the calibration is done, the technician must change attitudes—from engaging in a routinized operation to a careful cognitive inspection. The detection of an incorrect signal in one given channel during calibration requires that the technician change an improper setting or fix (or have fixed) this defective channel before proceeding. The calibration procedure should be viewed by technicians as *their test* to determine if the machine is ready for recording and not as a procedure directed by and for the electroencephalographer.

The same point made for the machine calibration must also be made for the patient calibration, a similar procedure, but with the patient (and some additional circuits) now included into the recording system. All channels record from the same linkage, often F_p1 to O1 or F_p2 to O2, to see if all channels are recording exactly the same way, as they should if the same linkage is recorded on each channel. The technician must now look carefully at each channel and make certain that all are the same with regard both to frequency and to amplitude. If one channel shows rhythms higher or lower in amplitude than the others, failure to notice this difference may mean that the recording will begin with one channel at a different amplification or filter setting than the others or with some defect affecting the amplification.

Waking Record

Make certain that a definite waking record is obtained. There are mainly two types of EEG abnormality: (1) slow waves and (2) sharp waves or spikes. Spikes often need a sleep record to appear, and slow waves usually need a wake record. Many slow waves will become indistinct or even disappear in a drowsy or sleep record and require a waking record before they clearly appear. Technicians should not allow their patients to become drowsy during the waking portion of the record by failing to monitor the state of their patients. Abnormal slow waves may then be missed. Technicians may complain that they cannot keep their patients awake for one part of the record, but they must not give sleep medication (such as chloral hydrate) at a time when its effectiveness is at the same time as the desired waking record. Also, various tactics can be used to keep the patient awake. Maintaining open eyes for a long period of time and using various forms of stimulation and encouragement will usually keep the patient sufficiently awake to obtain a satisfactory waking record.

One important point is that a waking record is better obtained *before* a sleep tracing than *after* the patient has been in stage II sleep. There are at least two problems with "waking" records obtained after sleep. One problem is the difficulty and, at times, the impossibility of arousing patients into a definite, full waking state *after* they have been soundly sleeping. All of us have experienced this same problem in ourselves or others after awakening from a sound sleep. The second problem that arises from trying to obtain the waking record after sleep is one that is not well known. The problem is that wakefulness, appropriately defined as showing clear alpha rhythms on the EEG and a responsiveness on the part of the patient, may not show the same rhythms right after sleep as before sleep. Certain waveforms may appear only immediately after awakening and look like an "abnormality," if one assumes a definite wakefulness on the part of the patient. An excellent example can be found in the form of occipital slow waves, seen especially in young patients. A comparison of the amount of occipital slow waves seen in the clear waking record (with alpha) *before* and *after* sleep will often reveal an excessive amount only *after* sleep. The electroencephalographer must judge the amount of this slowing to determine if it is excessive (and therefore abnormal). Often the amount in wakefulness *after* sleep is excessive by any standards and the amount *before* sleep in the same patient is an amount acceptable as normal. In particular, *before* sleep only slow transients may be seen, but *after* sleep the slowing may be high amplitude, rhythmical delta waves, considered excessive by most electroencephalographers. The clinical correlate of this important point may be that immediately after awakening from a sleep most subjects or patients are not as alert (although clearly awake) as they are before any drowsiness has occurred. The excessive occipital slow waves may be the EEG expression of this fact. If the only waking record available to the electroencephalographer is a segment recorded after a sleep, misleading patterns may appear. Waking records should thus be recorded as much as possible before and not after sleep tracings.

Filters

Avoid low linear frequency (LLF) = 5 (i.e., very short time constant) during the waking record. The setting of LLF = 5 should be used only under special circumstances. This setting indicates that the frequencies under 5/sec will nearly all be filtered out by the EEG machine; if this setting is used in the *waking* record when we are looking for slow waves, most of the slowing in the EEG will be filtered out and therefore never appear. Although technicians may "clean up" a record by reducing or eliminating the very slow waves, especially from movement or electrode artifacts, they have also eliminated the important information contained in the waking record. This latter point emphasizes the reason why technicians are tempted to use a short time constant (LLF = 5) in waking records; they convert a very messy record full of artifacts to a cleaner, more attractive one, but they also eliminate crucial information.

Only a few circumstances permit the use of the setting LLF = 5. One situation is during a sleep record, which will be searching for spikes or sharp waves, after a satisfactory waking record has already been obtained. If some type of slow artifact develops at that time (from perspiration or a loose electrode) and the considered judgment of the technician is that fixing the artifact will awaken the patient who will not likely fall asleep again, then this setting may be justified. The sharp waves or spikes will then appear clearly, if they exist, and elimination of the slow wave components of the sleep record may not be too misleading. This latter procedure, however, should be considered a last-resort maneuver, since the goal of each recording is to look at all the rhythms that are there. Other instances that may permit the use of short time constants for a *portion* of the EEG include records with both very slow and fast activity (especially in a comatose patient); the elimination of the very slow activity may then allow for a more clear assessment of the remaining fast activity.

Artifacts

Fix an electrode that is obviously producing artifacts. Part of the training of an EEG technician is to teach a certain philosophical approach to EEG technology. The approach to avoid is the passive attitude, as if the technician were on the sidelines watching the events that transpired. With this attitude untrained technicians may make a token attempt to fix a bad electrode, but if unsuccessful the first time, they may quickly move on to another montage that does not use that particular faulty electrode. Trained EEG technicians usually have developed not a passive but an active attitude, characterized by the commitment to obtain a good record by whatever means necessary. These technicians assume the responsibility of providing the electroencephalographer with the best possible tracing, and they will use all of their expertise and energy to correct every possible defect. If an electrode is producing artifacts, they immediately clean again the area where it was attached, clean the electrode and examine it, and then reapply it. If this same electrode still produces artifacts, the technician will likely replace it with one that works satisfactorily. The appropriate attitude is to pursue until the artifacts are gone, knowing that the recording can be and will be done correctly.

Hyperventilation

Carefully monitor and evaluate how well the hyperventilation (HV) is performed by the patient. HV is an important activating procedure and may come at the time when the patient (who may have been sleep deprived and/or given some mild sedative) has difficulty staying awake. This activating procedure seems to have one of two extreme effects on many patients—producing either an agitation or the opposite, a drowsiness. If the latter effect appears, a sleep deprived patient, whose HV further brings on drowsiness, may be sound asleep when the technician believes HV is occurring. The deep breathing characteristic of certain sleep stages may mimic the exaggerated respiration that has been requested. The important point here is that the technician should be watching the EEG record and should be able to tell the difference between the diffuse slowing (build-up) of HV and the diffuse slowing of sleep. When sleep spindles are seen during the time when the patient is supposed to be hyperventilating and the technician evaluates the HV effort as excellent, then neither the patient's effort nor the EEG tracing was being examined. When the HV comes at the end of an EEG after a sleep tracing, the patient is then often drowsy and can easily fall back to sleep during this procedure. Proper comparison of two records taken at different times from the same patient, showing abnormalities during HV, depends on a similar *effort* used to perform the hyperventilation; therefore, the technician should always evaluate this effort.

Montage

Designate a new montage, but always remember to change the master switch to this montage on the EEG machine. Most EEG machines have preset runs, that is, a switch that includes all of the prewired montages that are ordinarily used on all patients, and a simple change of this dial will allow the technician to move on to the next routine electrode combination. When the time for a new montage arrives, most technicians follow a certain routine, for example, draw in the run on a head diagram imprinted on the EEG paper, then designate the gain and the filter settings and finally change the montage switch. If the attention of the technicians is diverted between the last two operations, they may then forget to turn the switch, so the new run is designated on the record, but in actuality is the previous run continued. This mistake occurs enough to make a point of it. The solution to this problem is the same as in most of these situations; the technician should always carefully watch the record and hopefully will pick up the fact that the distribution of the rhythms appears wrong for this new run. If that judgment is not made (and it can be a difficult judgment for many technicians and for some electroencephalographers) when the next montage comes up, the technician should then have noticed an incorrect designation on the montage dial. The correct procedure for the technician at this point after this mistake is, of course, not to move onto the next montage and hope that the electroencephalographer will never discover the problem, but to acknowledge the mistake. The incorrectly labeled run should then be properly designated and the montage that was skipped should be dialed and run.

Seizure

Keep the EEG machine running at the onset of a clinical seizure. The rhythms that are recorded at the beginning of a clinical seizure are by far the most significant information that an electroencephalographer can obtain on a patient with epilepsy. The interictal sharp waves or spikes are very significant, but the ictal activity during the attack itself conveys the most important information, namely, which area in the brain is responsible for the clinical attacks. If a technician turns off the EEG machine just while these rhythms are developing, the most crucial information obtainable on that patient has been eliminated. The problem is not that technicians have concluded that turning off the machine is the best maneuver, but this action seems almost reflexive on the part of some technicians. They see or hear some disturbance from the patient and two appropriate tendencies then unfold: (1) turn off the machine so the artifact that usually appears does not swamp out the recording and (2) move into the patients' room to see what can be done for them. Since the action to turn off the recording is nearly a reflex, the best way to avoid the problem is to acknowledge that there will be a great temptation to turn off the record, and then, with this caution in mind, forever guard against doing just that with encouraging reminders from the electroencephalographer.

Sleep Record

Make certain to obtain a sleep record on patients with episodic symptoms, possible or clear seizure disorders. The major use of an EEG machine in most laboratories is to uncover or confirm a seizure disorder. The majority of patients with epilepsy will require a sleep record to show their interictal sharp wave, spike, or spike-wave activity. Only patients with an active focus demonstrate these discharges in a waking record; therefore, sleep tracings are extremely important in any EEG lab. Unfortunately, the economic and fiscal pressures in some laboratories have put too great an emphasis on doing more records per day, and sleep tracings, of course, reduce this number. An EEG without a sleep tracing on a patient with epilepsy, however, may reveal as little as a plain skull film in a patient with a rapidly growing glioma. Slow transients or slow waves, even those appearing in the waking record in some "paroxysmal" way, do not confirm a seizure disorder; as interictal events only spikes, spike and wave complexes, or sharp waves can confirm an epilepsy and these discharges usually require a sleep tracing.

The success of obtaining a sleep tracing on all patients with possible or definite epilepsy is dependent on a number of factors. Clear instructions to the patient before the appointment should include the need to be sleep deprived (50% of their usual sleep), resulting not only in an increased probability to obtain sleep during the EEG, but also an increased chance that a focus, if present, will be more active. The rest of the routine of the patient *on the day of the test* should not be disturbed; medication and meals should be taken as usual, but *no* stimulating beverage with caffeine (coffee, tea, carbonated drinks, etc.) should be drunk prior to the test. Before the preparation of the patient, he or she should be asked if a bathroom is required and, during the record, he or she should be made as comfortable as possible. At times, soft music can also be of value in helping patients to relax and to sleep. The technician should now use good judgment to obtain an acceptable sleep record. A quick, but unsuccessful, 15- to 20-minute attempt is not acceptable. A second dose of sleep medication can usually be safely given 30 to 35 minutes after the first unsuccessful dose, and the technician should also inquire into any problems that the patient may be experiencing in achieving sleep. Of course, there are a certain *small* number of patients who will not or cannot sleep in an EEG lab, but each technician should try everything possible to obtain a sleep record, especially on those patients with episodic symptoms. One good rule in all EEG labs is that sleep should be obtained on all patients with epilepsy and should at least be attempted on all other patients, since this stage often brings unexpected information—data of the most useful kind.

Photic Stimulation

Do photic stimulation while the patient is awake. Photic stimulation is performed on patients mainly for two reasons: (1) to compare the photic driving responses on the two sides of the head to see if one side is significantly depressed (see Figure 5.4) and (2) to attempt to elicit epileptiform activity, usually of a generalized, corticoreticular type (bilateral spike and wave complexes). The procedure takes only a short time, requires relatively inexpensive equipment, and is invaluable in certain cases, especially in those who show bilaterally synchronous and symmetrical spike and wave complexes *only* during photic stimulation and not at any other time. This reviewer is convinced that there are far fewer patients in the USA in 1993 with a photoconvulsive response of bilateral spike and wave complexes to light flashes, compared to the 3% of all patients with an EEG who showed such a response in the late 1950s. It seems possible that the many examples of flickering lights in our society may be responsible for a partial adaptation to these photic flashes.

Photic flashes at different frequencies (e.g., 1, 3, 6, 9, 12, 15, 18, 21, and 24/sec) should be presented to the patients while they are *awake,* when photic driving and epileptiform responses *more likely will appear.* In many laboratories a sleep record is routinely done before the photic stimulation. When a patient has just awakened, this waking state may be difficult to maintain, but a definite attempt should be made to keep the patient fully awake during photic stimulation to increase the chances of photic driving or spike and wave complexes. Obviously some patients, such as uncooperative children, would best be stimulated photically in a sleep state if they had earlier been uncooperative in the waking state.

Cleaning Patient

Make certain that electrode paste or marking pencil is removed from the scalp of the patient. This point should require little comment, but occasionally even good technicians can be careless in trying to rush on to the next patient, leaving paste or grease pencil marks on the last one. Patients (or their families) have very few ways to judge an EEG laboratory, and one of those few ways is to check on how well the scalp is cleaned after the test. An excellent record, done with great expertise, proper activating procedures, and accurate localization and interpretation, will not make the reputation of that EEG laboratory from the *patient's point of view.* Patients know only how they are handled and prepared before and after the recording.

Spilling Liquids on EEG Machine

Carefully guard against the spilling of any kind of fluid on the EEG machine. Coffee, tea, and other beverages can be conveniently placed on the EEG machine at any time. Spilling the contents of any liquid down into the machine can cause expensive repairs, and this possibility must be absolutely avoided. In the few instances in which the author has known this to have occurred, a visitor to the lab (transporter, student nurse) was the one who actually spilled the liquid, but the *technician* was the one who placed the beverage on the machine. The only safe rule is *never* to place a container of any liquid on the EEG machine; although the EEG personnel may be careful not to spill it, others may not be so careful.

Common Problems Between the Referring Physician and the EEG Laboratory

Relevant History

Provide as much relevant history as possible on the EEG requisition. These data are not so much for the purposes of providing research material but to permit the running of an EEG recording utilizing the best of strategies. For example, if clinical signs and symptoms (e.g., an aphasia) exist, then extra montages emphasizing the left frontal and temporal areas can be run. If sensorimotor disorders are evident, then parasagittal montages can be emphasized, rather than temporal ones. Finally, if episodic symptoms are included in the patient's history, then every effort should be made to obtain a sleep tracing to maximize the chances of recording any possible epileptiform activity. The referring physician may also ask on the EEG requisition specific questions of the electroencephalographer, who can either (1) answer those questions within the formal report or (2) attach a separate note to the EEG report as an informal comment.

Permission for Hyperventilation

Indicate permission for hyperventilation. The three major contraindications for HV are (1) recent cardiac disorders, such as a myocardial infarction, (2) respiratory diseases, and (3) sickle cell disease. The reason for avoiding HV in the first two instances is obvious, but for patients with sickle cell disease a conservative approach is preferred to avoid any possible sickle cell crisis during the hyperventilation.

Permission for Photic Stimulation

Specify any contraindication to photic stimulation. Many laboratories routinely stimulate each patient photically, and only those patients whose seizures are easily activated by flickering lights need to be especially identified on the EEG requisition. In these cases the photic stimulation should still likely be done, if permitted by the patient, to verify a photic sensitivity, as information of great importance. The photic stimuli, however, can be presented very carefully by the technician, who can immediately cease the stimulation at the moment epileptiform activity appears on the EEG tracing. With prior warning of possible photosensitivity, the chances of driving even a photically sensitive patient into a clinical attack should be minimal. This reviewer knows of a patient who had a generalized tonic-clonic seizure (GTC) during photic stimulation in an EEG laboratory, fell off the cart, broke a shoulder, and sued everyone involved. Although the suit was unsuccessful, the important point is that the technician must be ready to stop the flashes at the moment that epileptiform activity first appears in the EEG to avoid a GTC seizure.

Permission for Sleep Medication

Provide permission for sleep medication, such as chloral hydrate. Obviously, any history of drug sensitivity should be included on the requisition, as should any comments relating to the chances of the patient's sleeping in the laboratory with the aid of medication. If the patient is known to be an insomniac with a history of difficulty in falling asleep at any time, this information helps the electroencephalographer to advise the technician regarding the appropriate dose of the sleep medication. If a patient must return for a second (sleep) tracing at a later time, because of an unsuccessful attempt to sleep, he or she will likely be upset, and the referring physician must then wait for a longer time for a full report.

Verbal Report

Request a summarized verbal report by telephone in special cases. Most electroencephalographers are willing to provide a verbal EEG report to physicians who require this information to make some immediate decision regarding their patient. Questions concerning possible (1) status epilepticus or (2) brain death usually require an immediate EEG interpretation and then verbal communication to the referring physician. Also, the EEG report on any patient with (unsuspected) severe electrographic abnormalities should be quickly transmitted to be as helpful as possible to the clinician. Generally, if the referring physician considers an immediate EEG report necessary for any given patient, then the electroencephalographer should respect the justified need for this information and provide the verbal report, in addition to the formal typed report that follows.

The Medicolegal EEG

We now live in the world of litigation, and all electroencephalographers must be prepared to testify in a court of law regarding EEGs they have interpreted. We may find ourselves in court to testify as expert witnesses in cases of head injury, with or without possible post-traumatic epilepsy, and also when a seizure disorder is a possible contributing factor in a given crime. Furthermore, an electroencephalographer may be called on to provide evidence regarding the possible incompetency or legal insanity of a patient.

Mental Incompetency Versus Insanity

The tests for incompetency refer to an inability on the part of the individual charged with an offense (1) to understand the nature and purpose of the proceedings against him or her, (2) to assist in his or her defense, and (3) to understand the nature and purpose of any sentence that may be imposed by a court of law. Insanity is a legal term and refers to the inability on the part of the individual charged with a crime to understand the difference between right and wrong. Electroencephalographers may be called to present evidence that may argue for one or the other condition.

M'Naghten Rules

A defendant cannot be held responsible for an act if he or she cannot comprehend the character of the act performed or, if comprehending, he or she cannot chose between right and wrong. As Morse[180] points out, the term *comprehend* here refers to one of the M'Naghten Rules known as *cognition* and the word *choose* relates to another one of those rules known as *will*. Thus, the defendant may choose to do wrong if incapable of choosing to do right, and this is known as "uncontrollable impulse" or "irresistible impulse" in the traditional principles of legal insanity.

EEG as Legal Evidence

When electroencephalographers testify in court they will likely be asked to define the term *electroencephalogram*. Some states include within their legal statutes such a definition, as is found in Louisiana, which defined EEG as "graphic recording of the electrical currents developed in the cortex by brain action and by this examination it can be determined whether (a person) actually suffered any damage to his brain." There is usually no difficulty in introducing the EEG as legal evidence and a higher court (appellate) in Illinois ruled that EEG can thus be presented as evidence. At least one high court has decided that it is prejudicial to exclude EEGs when they are relevant. In this instance the appellate division of the Supreme Court in New York held that the EEG tracings and the interpretation thereof by a medical expert were admissible as evidence.

Woolsey and Goldner[181] have made some definite suggestions to electroencephalographers to ensure proper identification of an EEG record introduced into court. For example, they suggest that the EEG be marked at the time it is taken with the name and address of the patient, the place of the test, and the name of the technician. They point out that many courts will permit the introduction of the EEG through the testimony of the physician interpreting the record and that the technician need not be present. During that same conference Woolsey and Goldner point out that it is usually possible that both parties will stipulate regarding the authenticity and accuracy of the EEG record, but the reviewer has found that this latter point is usually a matter of considerable debate, examination, and cross-examination. Gibbs and Gibbs[182] have also made some excellent suggestions for electroencephalographers about to appear in court. For example, they suggest that a recording that *likely* will end up in a courtroom should not be cut down. The tracing should be continuous and, if possible, contained within a given pack of paper. They also suggest that the patient or guardian sign the EEG on the face of this recording, as soon as it is completed, in the presence of the technician. If a new pack of paper should be inserted into the EEG during the recording, this second pack should be numbered and identified and also signed by the patient or guardian. The technician should, of course, sign the recording in the presence of the patient or guardian. All signatures should appear on the face of the recording together with the date and all the pertinent information related to the recording. On the question of the necessity of the electroencephalographer's presence at the time the EEG was taken, the electroencephalographer should be prepared to be challenged as to his or her possible absence during the actual recording. A simple statement, however, will usually suffice; it should explain that physicians are generally not present for any of these recordings, which are taken by technicians under their *supervision*.

Head Injury

The most typical example of an instance in which the electroencephalographer will be called to testify in court is in the question of a significant head injury. One of the major problems in assessing the significance of any abnormal EEG pattern in a patient who has suffered a head injury is that very rarely do electroencephalographers have evidence of the status of the EEG prior to the head injury. Therefore, the electroencephalographer must use statistical probabilities based on previous evidence and experience to judge the likelihood that any given abnormality may be the result of a head injury. Gibbs and his colleagues as early as 1944[183] provided some statistics that could be of value in this instance. For example, the general conclusion was drawn that a focal EEG abnormality in patients with head trauma strongly suggested the presence of "brain damage"; more specifically, if a generalized abnormality was present 3 months or more after a mild head injury, the chances were 6 to 1 that the abnormality antedated the head injury. If the EEG was normal, the chances were 53 to 8 that the patient did not have post-traumatic epilepsy. Finally, if a paroxysmal abnormality was noted, the chances were 27 to 2 that the patient had some type of epileptic condition. If the patient had clinical seizures and a focal paroxysmal abnormality more than 3 months after a head injury, the chances (according to the authors) were considered to be 21 to 7 that those seizures were the result of the trauma rather than the result of some other factor. These probabilities, of course, are based on statistics of that particular study and are useful in making intelligent judgments and predictions. These data were reported nearly 50 years ago and need to be updated; also, some conclusions remain speculative, as exemplified by the probability that a given focal abnormality is the result of a head injury.

Courjon[184] summarized the same kinds of probabilities (but less specific) based on more recent evidence. His general conclusion was that if an EEG is normal or shows only a very mild abnormality immediately after a head injury and continues to show a normal tracing, an organic lesion, of course, is very unlikely, but still is possible. On the other hand, long-lasting EEG abnormalities with slow abatement are characteristic of major organic cerebral injuries. The secondary deterioration of an EEG suggests either post-traumatic complications, such as a subdural hematoma, abscess, or seizures, or nontraumatic disease. In these instances complementary clinical investigations are, of course, definitely required. Persistent EEG abnormalities without any abatement suggest the same two possibilities, namely, post-traumatic complications or nontraumatic disease. If an EEG is performed *early* in the post-traumatic stage, there are usually good correlations between the clinical signs and the EEG abnormality, according to Jung.[185] If the EEG is done only *late* in the post-traumatic stage, the electroencephalographer is often asked to state the degree of probability that the head injury was the etiology of the abnormality, but this decision is difficult. One can, however, help to determine the extent of abnormality and locate nontraumatic brain lesions and predict the possibility of late post-traumatic complications.[186] According to Courjon, late EEGs cannot verify subjective symptoms such as headaches, dizziness, and post-traumatic psychiatric disturbances by an abnormal EEG, nor is it possible from a normal tracing to disprove the presence of those same symptoms. On the other hand, a normal EEG in the face of clear neurological deficits suggests that further clinical recovery is not expected.[187] If the EEG is normal, this normal pattern cannot guarantee that seizures will not occur,[188,189] and if the EEG is abnormal, this may be a clue for the development of late complications, especially seizures.

A spike or sharp wave focus at the site of the original traumatic lesion usually is associated with late epilepsy, but, of course, some patients never develop clinical seizures even with a persistent irritative EEG pattern in the form of a spike or sharp wave focus. If clear seizures do exist (except for the "petit mal" or absence type), the EEG can assist in determining the etiology.[190] For example, 3/sec spike and wave complexes in an adult are not usually compatible with post-traumatic epilepsy.[191]

Courjon[184] has also pointed out that two patterns in the EEG are often suspected as a post-traumatic pattern, namely (1) low voltage records and (2) posterior theta rhythms. Meyer-Mickeleit,[192] however, found low voltage EEGs in the normal population as often as in chronic head injuries, as did Scherzer[193] for posterior theta rhythms. Vogel[194] found that both of these patterns usually could be considered an inherited variant of cerebral activity. These studies argue strongly that low voltage patterns and posterior theta activity cannot necessarily be attributed to head injury.

Post-Traumatic Epilepsy

One important question is the duration of time after a head injury when post-traumatic epilepsy may first reveal itself. Based on his extensive legal (not medical) experience in personal injury suits, the renowned attorney Melvin M. Belli[195] has claimed that post-traumatic epilepsy may not show itself for as long as 18 years after the injury. Certainly, when time intervals of that magnitude are considered, head injury can usually be considered no more than a presumptive etiology for any type of seizure disorder. As in all other aspects of medicine and its related fields, probabilities are the tools of the physician making predictions or prognostications, and these prognoses are based on the statistics that have been collected on a particular issue. For example, Phillips[196] has provided statistics on the cumulative percentage of patients with post-traumatic epilepsy, according to the duration of time following the head injury. For example, in 3 months, 55% of those who will develop post-traumatic epilepsy will have manifested clinical seizures by that time. In 1 year 82% will have shown their seizures; in 2 years, 85%; and in 4 years, 97%. According to Phillips, by 11 years all patients developing seizures following a head injury will have shown some type of clinical seizure within that period of time. Jasper and Penfield[197] have provided slightly different statistics showing that 46% will have shown a seizure within 1 year, 63% in 3 years, and 80% within a 5-year period. More recently, Jennett[198] has reported an incidence of 56%, 77%, and 85% in 1, 3, and 5 years respectively. Ascroft[199] pointed out many years ago that penetration of the dura from a head injury is crucial for the determination of post-traumatic epilepsy. For example, in these latter studies 45% of those with dural penetration developed post-traumatic epilepsy, but if the dura had not been penetrated, only 23% showed seizures.

Perr[200] has concluded that the incidence of seizures after head injury varies from as low as 0.1% to as high as 50% depending on the investigation reviewed. Perr has also pointed out that idiopathic epilepsy is 15 to 20 times more common than post-traumatic seizures, and this one statistic provides some perspective on the relative incidence of post-traumatic epilepsy. The reviewer, however, would urge the reader to accept the latter statistics with caution since careful histories of patients with epilepsy seem to reduce the incidence of genuine "idiopathic" epilepsy, which may be less common than once thought. As one other negative point regarding the incidence of post-traumatic epilepsy, Hyslop[201] studied 715 head injuries introduced for litigation and the number of frankly fraudulent cases outnumbered the true cases of post-traumatic epilepsy by more than 2 to 1. Only 8.6% of these cases raised a reasonable possibility of post-traumatic epilepsy and only 20% of those latter instances could actually be verified.

Another important factor in the probability of seizures developing after head injury is the presence of an intracranial hematoma, which increases the incidence of early epilepsy from 4% to 27% and of late epilepsy from 3% to 35%.[198]

EEG Abnormality in Criminals

A number of EEGs have been done on criminals to determine if such individuals have an increased incidence of abnormal patterns. For example, in 1943 Silverman[202] found that prisoners showed a 53% incidence of EEG abnormality, but 2 years later Gibbs and his colleagues[203] in a larger group of prisoners found no particular deviation or disturbance in the EEG. On the other hand, Kennard et al.[204] in 1955 reported a greater incidence of abnormal EEGs in "criminal psychopaths" than in controls. Hill and Pond[205] wrote that slightly more than one-half of accused murderers had an abnormal EEG and during the same year Hill[206] published a more specific report on murderers, claiming excessive theta activity in 22% of these cases and posterior temporal slow wave activity in 8%, percentages greater than those found in the controls.

Some authors have reported a relatively low incidence of EEG abnormality among prisoners. One example is the report of Winkler and Kove[207] on prisoners with a homicidal history in whom only 24% were said to have an abnormal record and a similar study by Levy and Kennard[208] revealed only a 15% incidence. Small[209] reported on individuals who had committed felonies and found an EEG abnormality in only 33%.

A very high incidence of EEG abnormality has also been reported among criminals. For example, Stafford-Clark and Taylor[210] reported on murderers and found that 73% of them showed an abnormal EEG, especially in motiveless crimes. This value contrasted with a 25% incidence of abnormality among the controls in prison.[211] In that latter study an 83% incidence of abnormal EEGs was found in aggressive psychopaths in prison. Silverman[212] reported a 75% incidence of EEG abnormality, especially in those who had committed psychopathic crimes. Williams[213] reported a study of prisoners with repetitive assaultive behavior, compared to those who had committed only a single act of assault, and found that the former group had a significantly higher incidence of abnormal EEGs than those whose crime was only a single act. Similarly, Levy[214] found the incidence of EEG abnormality in recidivists to be twice as high as in persons who were imprisoned for the first time. In 1950 Alström[215] reported on 345 male epileptics and compared that group to 42,000 males in the general population with regard to the incidence of these latter two groups in the penal register. The register included 7.0% of the epileptics and 4.8% of males in the general population, suggesting that males with epilepsy may more frequently find themselves behind bars than other males. Among those in the penal register, violent crimes were committed by 17% of those with seizures, compared to 11% in the general population, but Alström was careful to point out that no crimes were apparently committed during a seizure.

The topic of abnormal EEGs in criminals introduces the idea that violent behavior may be the result of brain damage. This is not to say, however, that all violence is caused by individuals with damaged brains but that all behavior filters through the central nervous system, as is pointed out by Mark and Ervin.[216] These authors also point out that experiments have indicated that there is a definable neural system that organizes affective and directive attack behavior and that this system is linked to the limbic brain.

Mark and Ervin claim that chromosomal studies help to provide evidence that organicity may be involved with such violent behavior. For example, they claim that those with XXY chromosomes frequently show behavioral disorders and those with an XYY chromosomal pattern more frequently show such antisocial behavior. According to the review of Mark and Ervin, the (XY) siblings of those with an XYY pattern usually do not have a record of breaking the law, but the sibling of the XY inmates are frequently in jail. This general point would suggest that the *environment* of the inmates with the XY chromosomal pattern plays a very important role, while it is the specific abnormal *chromosomal pattern* in the XYY individuals that accounts in large part for the antisocial behavior.

Some studies suggest that the incidence of EEG abnormality may vary according to the nature of the crime. In the study by Stafford-Clark and Taylor,[210] those who had committed motivated murder under considerable provocation had a 17% incidence of abnormal EEG, similar to the incidence in the general population, and those who had murdered accidentally while committing some other felony showed a slightly higher incidence at 25%. These values contrast with those in explosive psychopaths who committed murder without motive, among whom 73% showed abnormal EEGs. The highest incidence was 86%, found among those who were obviously insane at the time they committed their crimes. These latter studies do suggest that a higher incidence of EEG abnormality is related to an increasing degree of violent (perhaps insane) behavior. Furthermore, in a study conducted by Walton[217] the EEGs of murderers were studied and 35% of those individuals had an abnormal EEG. Although lower than most groups studied in the previous report, this was a higher incidence than was found in those committing other kinds of crimes or in the general population. As Curran[218] has emphasized, however, the possession of an abnormal EEG might thus become a criminal asset and it is important for all electroencephalographers to keep this point in mind. An abnormal EEG, of course, does not necessarily constitute proof of the existence of epilepsy as an extenuating factor in a crime.

Possible Relationship of Temporal Lobe Epilepsy to Violence

These latter sections have emphasized the relationship of certain abnormal EEG findings to criminal behavior, and one specific possibility representing a most difficult problem is the relationship of epilepsy to violent behavior. Mark and Ervin[216] have pointed out that the symptoms of some temporal lobe seizures are very similar to those that precede episodes of aggression in violent individuals. In these instances, however, the latter authors agree that they are not seizures in the usual sense, because there is usually no loss of consciousness and no loss of memory for this violent behavior. On the other hand, the episodic violence is said to reflect a functional abnormality within the temporal lobe. Patients with temporal lobe abnormalities often share certain behavioral difficulties, including episodes of violence, and most of the individuals studied by Mark and Ervin suffered both from seizures and from violent episodes. Although temporal lobe epilepsy may be an important example of a known disease state that can be related to violent behavior, these authors are quick to point out that this does not mean that all temporal lobe epileptics are violent. Their belief is that temporal lobe disease can cause a number of conditions, including seizures, severe memory loss, speech difficulties, and poor impulse control, including violent behavior. It is the underlying malfunctioning of the limbic brain that is causally related to the poor impulse control and the violent behavior. The temporal lobe seizures represent *only one* symptom of a malfunctioning limbic system, and another symptom may be violent behavior.

Walker (*EEG and the Law*[219]) has outlined six criteria that are required to establish that a given crime may have been committed as a manifestation of a seizure: (1) the patient has bona fide epileptic abnormalities, (2) spontaneous attacks are similar to the one that occurred at the time of the crime, (3) the period of the loss of awareness and (4) degree of assumed unconsciousness are commensurate with the type of epileptic attack usually experienced by the patient or defendant, (5) the EEG findings are compatible with a seizure disorder, and (6) the circumstances are compatible with the assumption of the lack of awareness of the individual at the time of the crime. These six criteria are usually very difficult, if not impossible, to meet in violent crimes said to (possibly) be related to a seizure disorder. Furthermore, Sir Norwood East (see Walton[217]) has pointed out that murders are rarely ever committed even after an epileptic seizure during a post-ictal stage when behavior, possibly called violent, could occur. Walton[217] has summarized the evidence for murder during a seizure as scanty and states that an epileptic discharge in the EEG does not provide sufficient grounds to support a defense of diminished responsibility unless there are clear clinical grounds to support a disturbance of consciousness during the act. Furthermore, Lennox[220] has summarized his 35 years of experience in epilepsy and has indicated that he was aware of only two instances of murder by patients with epilepsy and neither of these patients committed their crimes in any relationship to their seizures. Earlier in 1950 Alström[215] had reported that 17% of males with seizures who had been in the penal register had committed violent crimes, but none of these crimes had been committed during a seizure.

One example of a crime committed during a *possible* seizure was portrayed in a moot trial by the Southern EEG Society in a volume entitled *Electroencephalography and the Law.*[219] In this instance the jury apparently was not convinced that a temporal lobe epilepsy could explain violent behavior and thus exonerate the defendant.

Other similar cases have been reported in the courts of this country. For example, as early as 1895 in a case decided by the United States Court of Appeals for the District of Columbia, the accused entered a plea of not guilt by reason of "insanity." Reasoning comprising the defense was: (1) a number of psychomotor seizures had caused a state of insanity, (2) a seizure had caused a change of latent insanity to active insanity, and (3) the criminal act had actually transpired during a seizure. The court rejected the defense on the grounds that there was no evidence that the state of a seizure (or activated insanity) adhered to the M'Naghten rules required for the judicial recognition of insanity.

The term *automatism* has also found its way into the courts and was defined by the Court of Criminal Appeal in Northern Ireland in 1961. Automatism was considered the state wherein a person, though capable of action, "is not conscious of what he is doing. . . . It means unconscious involuntary action and it is a defense because the mind does not go with what is being done. . . ." Furthermore, automatism "means an act which is done by the muscles without any control by the mind such as a spasm, reflex action or a convulsion; or an act done by a person who is not conscious of what he is doing."

Morse[180] has pointed out that when a criminal act is committed during a psychomotor seizure there may be another kind of problem of legal responsibility; this may be relatively simple if the individuals with epilepsy have had at least one prior seizure, which establishes previous knowledge on the part of the patients of a condition which may have significant legal complications for them, rather than providing them with a ready defense. A case in point is *Smith v. Commonwealth* in a decision by the Court of Appeals in Kentucky in 1954. A person with epilepsy was prosecuted for manslaughter in the operation of an automobile. The defense was that the accused ran over a pedestrian due to a lapse of consciousness experienced as the result of a psychomotor seizure. In this case the court held that, whether or not the accused displayed willful indifference to the safety of other individuals by operating an automobile with such knowledge that he had epilepsy, constituted the important question of fact for the determination of the jury. Although conviction was reversed because of various kinds of errors in jury instruction a subsequent *conviction was affirmed* by the court of appeals of Kentucky in 1955.

Other cases have established diminished legal responsibility on the part of the driver with seizures. Such a case was the *People v. Freeman*, decided by the District Court of Appeal in California in 1943. The *Freeman* decision added an additional point that consideration should be given to the question of whether or not at the time the accused took to the highway in his automobile his epileptic condition permitted him to be fully aware and cognizant of what he was doing. If the answer was in the negative, then, according to the *Freeman* decision, the accused should not be held accountable. As Morse has pointed out, the sum and substance of the *Smith* decision seems to be that individuals with epilepsy who have had at least one prior seizure drive an automobile distinctly at their own criminal risk. According to Morse, the *Smith* decision may appear to be more reasonable than the *Freeman* decision since the safety of the public and the consideration for potential automobile accident victims should certainly outweigh the importance of a driving privilege for a person with epilepsy.

There are really very few instances in the world literature of crimes possibly committed during a clear clinical seizure. Perhaps a few cases presented by Mark and Ervin[216] in their book *Violence and the Brain* constitute evidence that a seizure state *might* exist during violent behavior. The most convincing evidence of the possible relationship of temporal lobe epilepsy to violent behavior is found in the case of Julia, who at one time attacked a girl with a sharp instrument and actually pierced the heart of that victim. Spikes were found on the temporal lobe during a routine EEG; with implanted electrodes Mark and Ervin recorded epileptic activity from both amygdalae. The stimulation of the amygdala resulted in symptoms like those seen at the beginning of the clinical seizures of this patient. In one instance clear seizure activity was recorded within the amygdala and at that time the patient got out of bed, ran to the wall, narrowed her eyes, bared her teeth, clenched her fists, and showed all the signs of being on the verge of launching an attack. Epileptic activity could be elicited as the result of electrical stimulation through these implanted electrodes, and rage behavior was often seen as the patient actually attacked the wall. At another time she smashed a guitar against the wall when "seizure-like" activity was found within the amygdala. At other times electrical stimulation of the amygdala initiated rage and violence, and this behavior was preceded by the development of local electrical seizure activity. The authors state that "there could be no doubt that the electrical stimulation of and the abnormal seizure activity from the amygdala preceded and was directly related to Julia's violence." This latter case represents one of the very few instances in the history of epileptology and criminology in which very *suggestive* evidence is brought to bear on this question of the possible direct relationship between temporal lobe epilepsy and violent behavior. The legal and medical communities, however, still await a *clear* example of a crime of violence committed during a *definite* seizure, as indicated by the conclusions of an international panel of epileptologists who found only 19 patients with "aggression."[221] This impressive study sampled 5,400 patients from 16 different epilepsy centers throughout the world and utilized simultaneous video-EEG monitoring on those patients with possible ictal violence. The most violent act that could be confirmed by EEG monitoring was the scratching of a face. There seems to be no more than a remote possibility that individuals having a complex partial seizure could direct their violence with the required full awareness of the environment to cause serious harm to another person. However, after the seizure during the post-ictal stage, the individual will likely have greater awareness of the environment but still be in a confusional state when crimes of violence could more likely occur.

Limitation of EEG in the Courtroom

Various degrees of pessimism have been expressed by a number of authors regarding the usefulness of the EEG in the courtroom. For example, Kiloh and Osselton[222] report that, in the field of forensic psychiatry, electroencephalography, with its shades of value and relatively low scale of probability, finds little application. They point to two cases of murder discussed by Curran.[218] In both of these cases EEG showed quite obvious abnormalities—one case with spike and wave activity and the other with changes that were suggestive of a localized brain lesion. There was no clinical evidence, however, to support a diagnosis of epilepsy in either one and in both cases the crimes seemed to be described as calculated and purposive. It was argued at both of the trials that the EEG abnormalities indicated the presence of "brain pathology" relevant to the commission of the crimes. As Kiloh and Osselton point out, these arguments were discarded by both juries and subsequent necropsy of the brain in each case proved to be normal. On the other hand, it should be emphasized that many individuals with epilepsy have thorough neuropathological examinations with negative results; the negative clinical histories would seem to be more significant than the negative necropsy.

Perr[200] has summarized the evidence on this matter of the limitations of EEG in the courtroom and finds that the EEG data following injury are of little prognostic significance and this general statement must make electroencephalographers cautious about their predictions in a court of law. Furthermore, Walton[217] has indicated that he had given up using EEG in medicolegal cases. He did point out, however, that although a single EEG in head injury cases was of little diagnostic or prognostic value, the serial recordings were useful in expressing the likelihood of the development of post-traumatic epilepsy. Clinical experience, rather than the EEG alone, was what Walton relied on in these questions. On the other hand, this reviewer does not share the pessimism of these latter authors since he has participated in many trials in which EEG played a prominent and proper role. The recurring symposia at regional and national meetings on "legal EEG" also demonstrate that EEG continues to find its way into many court cases.

Practical Suggestions in Medicolegal Cases

In the publication of the moot trial by the Southern EEG Society, Samuel Little[219] summarized various suggestions for the electroencephalographer who will be testifying in court. First, he pointed out the extreme importance of good identification on each EEG tracing, since one never knows while the EEG is run whether or not a particular tracing will become part of the medicolegal proceeding, in which the identification might become a crucial matter. He also noted that this trial emphasized the importance of being certain about medications taken prior to the test and of performing both awake and sleep records, and the value of obtaining serial tracings whenever possible. The expert witnesses in this moot trial also referred to the importance of a flexible use of amplification or gain controls and the importance of taking into consideration the age of the patient in the interpretation of the record. These latter proceedings have also shown the technologists the necessity of extreme technical care and excellent calibration, the importance of keeping artifacts to a minimum, and the necessity of obtaining supplementary history from the patient. Little concluded that the electroencephalographer's report should not just feed back clinical information found in the medical record, but all the clinical data available should be integrated with EEG findings to produce a unified presentation.

Gibbs and Gibbs[182] offer some excellent suggestions for the electroencephalographer about to appear in court. They point out that the electroencephalographer may receive telephone calls from lawyers of both sides and from the patient or members of the family. In these instances, obviously the physician must be extremely careful about imparting information, especially to the "other side." Gibbs and Gibbs point out that legal proceedings are usually cumbersome and that the electroencephalographer may need to spend an entire day without being called to the stand. They further point out that on the succeeding day one may be forced to spend many more hours conveying a small amount of information that would have required only a few words if one were allowed to state them in a normal matter. It is one strong suggestion from this reviewer that the appointments made between the electroencephalographer and the lawyer for a court appearance should be made for the earliest possible hour in the morning, usually 10 o'clock. Under these circumstances one usually can get on the stand in the early morning, but if one waits for the afternoon for his scheduled first appearance, delays of the morning usually infringe on that time and one can usually count on a wait before being called to the witness stand.

Gibbs and Gibbs point out that science and law do not mix and that "lawsuits seem to be a survival from a prescientific era, a kind of trial by combat." They point out that both sides distort the evidence as much as they can and that the lawyers on both sides attempt to cajole, trick, or actually frighten the witnesses into saying what they do not mean to say. The reviewer would generally agree with these latter points. Also, Gibbs and Gibbs point out that lawyers commonly indulge in forms of unpleasantness that are rarely encountered outside a courtroom. Normal procedure in the court may also involve disparaging comments regarding the intelligence, competence, and probity of the witness; however, the reviewer would emphasize the role of the attorney responsible for the court appearance of the electroencephalographers in safeguarding their reputation. The Gibbses conclude that the electroencephalographers, if handled roughly, should not feel that they have been singled out for special abuse (nearly everyone may receive the same kind of treatment). Additional comments by this reviewer would be to indicate the importance of a pretrial discussion with the attorney who has called one to court. Each and every question to be asked of the electroencephalographer in court should be written out by the attorney and the answer to each of these questions should be clear to the electroencephalographer. The electroencephalographer often must instruct the attorney about the kinds of questions that the attorney should ask when those questions directly relate to the electroencephalogram. Many attorneys are somewhat knowledgeable in EEG, but most will require some help from the electroencephalographer in formulating good questions to prepare a case that a given record either is normal or shows specific abnormalities. Some advice that is regrettably given is that electroencephalographers should request that they be paid "on the spot" for their time in the pretrial conference; also, most expert witnesses require payment *before* testifying, especially if called by the prosecution in a personal injury suit. Most attorneys expect such a request, which does not invalidate the testimony to be given, in that physicians have a right to be paid for their time in court. There is one further comment by this reviewer which is very important. During cross-examination the electroencephalographer should try to foresee the direction the other (opposing) attorney is taking in cross-examination to avoid being led into traps. One should also be aware that a "yes" or "no" answer to questions can be misleading to everyone in the courtroom including the jury and, if the judgment is that yes-no answers are leading to incorrect conclusions, one should request permission from the judge to explain the answers in greater detail. The Gibbses also refer to this problem and point out that the electroencephalographer is asked to subscribe to the legal fiction that the truth can be extracted through questions that are answered simply "yes" or "no," but that one is required under oath to tell the *whole* truth and nothing but the truth. They also point out that electroencephalographers must be aware that their answers may be adding up to a total falsehood and that they should turn to the judge and indicate that they must be able to explain further and in greater detail. In the experience of this reviewer most judges will permit one to provide such details. As the Gibbses point out, neither the attorney for the plaintiff nor the attorney for the defense is really interested in the truth as the electroencephalographer sees it, but it is important for electroencephalographers to present the truth clearly, as they see it, in the most accurate way. These two authors also point out that there are various well-known "tricks" often used by most attorneys during cross-examination. These include statements that most brain wave abnormalities are really meaningless, either because they occur in persons who are perfectly normal or that they can be caused by "anything." Another usual "trick" is to declare the EEG inadmissible because the electroencephalographer did not *see* the patient at the time of the recording. Also, the usual absence of the electroencephalographer during the recording is another point that is usually brought out by the opposing attorney, but electroencephalographers must quickly add (whenever they can) that our presence is rarely ever required during most recordings. One of the most subtle tricks commonly utilized in cross-examination in this reviewer's experience is that the attorney will use terms that have questionable definitions and ask for agreement from the electroencephalographer regarding some statement incorporating those terms. After the witness has agreed that a number of these statements are correct, one may find that they add up to a conclusion opposite to the stated position. The important point here is to require and request a precise definition from the attorney when a term is used that has a questionable definition. This puts the attorneys on the defensive and reverses what they are trying to accomplish. The Gibbses point out that it is helpful to remember that the other attorney is going to try to "get your goat" and that supposedly there are no hard feelings afterwards.

The reviewer concludes this section by emphasizing the need for a positive attitude on the part of the electroencephalographer in court. If the attorney and electroencephalographer have carefully planned their scenario and each knows what the other will be saying, then the only problem that remains will be the cross-examination from the "opposing" attorney. Here a positive attitude is required in which electroencephalographers must forever be aware of their stated position in the case, must try to foresee how the other attorney is attempting to shake their testimony, and should *consider* these verbal interchanges as an interesting *intellectual challenge.* After all, we should know our business better than any attorney and should triumph in all or most of these intellectual combats, if remaining calm and cool. With a positive attitude of this sort, the reviewer has actually enjoyed some courtroom appearances, finding them to be fascinating experiences.

References

1. Report of the Committee on Methods of Clinical Examination in Electroencephalography. Electroencephalogr Clin Neurophysiol 1958; 10:370–75.
2. American Electroencephalographic Society. Guidelines in EEG, 1–7 (Revised 1985). J Clin Neurophysiol 1986; 3:131–68.
3. Kellaway P. An orderly approach to visual analysis: parameters of the normal EEG in adults and children. In: Klass DW, Daly DD, eds. Current practice of clinical electroencephalography. New York: Raven, 1979; 69–147.
4. Galin D, Ellis RR. Asymmetry in evoked potentials as an index of lateralized cognitive processes in relation to EEG alpha asymmetry. Neuropsychobiology 1975; 13:45–50.
5. Gibbs, FA, Knott JR. Growth of the electrical activity of the cortex. Electroencephalogr Clin Neurophysiol 1949; 1:223–29.
6. Obrist WD. The electroencephalogram of normal aged adults. Electroencephalogr Clin Neurophysiol 1954; 6:235–44.
7. Hubbard O, Sunde D, Goldensohn ES. The EEG in centenarians. Electroencephalogr Clin Neurophysiol 1976; 40:407–17.
8. Rechtschaffen A, Kales A. A manual of standardized terminology, technique and scoring system for sleep stages of human subjects. Washington, D.C.: Government Printing Office, 1968.
9. Dement WC. Daytime sleepiness and sleep "attacks." In: Guilleminault C, Dement WC, Passouant P, eds. Narcolepsy. New York: Spectrum, 1976.
10. Kales A, Bixler EO, Tan TL, Scharf MD, Kales JD. Chronic hypnotic drug use. Ineffectiveness, drug-withdrawal insomnia and dependence. JAMA 1974; 227:513–7.
11. Hughes JR, King BD, Cutter JA, Markello R. The EEG in hyperventilated, lightly anesthetized patients. Electroencephalogr Clin Neurophysiol 1962; 14:274–7.
12. Goldberg HH, Strauss H. Distribution of slow activity induced by hyperventilation. Electroencephalogr Clin Neurophysiol 1959; 11:615.
13. Davis H, Wallace WM. Factors affecting changes produced in electroencephalogram by standardized hyperventilation. Arch Neurol Psychiatry 1942; 47:606–25.
14. Kurtz D. The EEG in parathyroid dysfunction. I: Glaser GH, ed. Handbook of electroencephalography and clinical neurophysiology, (C.) metabolic, endocrine and toxic disease. Amsterdam: Elsevier, 1976; 77–87.

15. Hughes JR. Usefulness of photic stimulation in routine clinical electroencephalography. Neurology (Minneap) 1960; 10:777–82.

16. Dreyfus-Brisac C. The bioelectrical development of the central nervous system during early life. In: Falkner F, ed. Human development. New York: Saunders, 1966; 286–305.

17. Tharp BR. Neonatal and pediatric electroencephalography. In: Aminoff MJ, ed. Electrodiagnosis in clinical neurology. New York: Churchill Livingstone, 1980; 67–117.

18. Schulte FJ, Michaelis R, Nolte R, Albert G, Parl U, Lasson U. Brain and behavioral maturation in new-born infants of diabetic mothers. Part I. Nerve conduction and EEG patterns. Neuropaediatrie 1969; 1:24–35.

19. Dreyfus-Brisac C. Sleep ontogenesis in early human prematurity from 24 to 27 weeks of conceptual age. Dev Psychobiol 1968; 1:162–9.

20. Gibbs FA, Gibbs EL. Atlas of electroencephalography. Vol. IV. Normal and abnormal infants from birth to 11 months of age. Reading, Mass.: Addison-Wesley, 1978; 373 pp.

21. Dreyfus-Brisac C. Neonatal electroencephalography. In: Scarpelli EM, Cosmi EV, eds. Review in perinatal medicine. New York: Raven, 1979, 3:397–483.

22. Hughes JR, Fino J, Gagnon L. Periods of activity and quiescence in the premature EEG. Neuropaediatrie 1983; 14:66–72.

23. Hughes JR, Miller JK, Fino J, Hughes CA. The sharp theta rhythm on the occipital areas of prematures (STOP): A newly described waveform. Clin EEG 1990; 21(2):77–87.

24. Hughes JR, Fino J, Hart LA. Premature temporal theta (PTΘ). Electroencephalogr Clin Neurophysiol 1987; 67:7–15.

25. Monod N, Garma L. Auditory responsivity in the human premature. Bio Neonate (Basel) 1965; 8:281–307.

26. Dreyfus-Brisac C. Ontogenesis of sleep in human prematures after 32 weeks of conceptual age. Dev Psychobiol 1970; 3:91–121.

27. Watanabe K, Iwase K, Hara K. Development of slow wave sleep in low birth weight infants. Dev Med Child Neurol 1974; 16:23–31.

28. Prechtl HFR. The behavioral states of the new-born infants (a review). Brain Res 1974; 76:185–212.

29. Samson-Dollfus D. L'EEG du prématuré jusqu'à l'âge de 3 mois et du nouveau-né à term. In: Thèse med. Paris: Foulon, 1955; 160.

30. Parmelee AH. Changes in the sleep patterns in premature infants as a function of brain maturation. In: Minkowski A, ed. Regional development of the brain in early life. Oxford: Blackwell, 1967; 459–80.

31. Monod N, Pajot N, Guidasci S. The neonatal EEG: statistical studies and prognostic value in full-term and pre-term babies. Electroencephalogr Clin Neurophysiol 1972; 32:529–44.

32. Lombroso CT. Quantified electrographic scales on 10 pre-term healthy newborns followed up to 40–43 weeks of conceptual age by serial polygraphic recordings. Electroencephalogr Clin Neurophysiol 1979; 46:460–74.

33. Lombroso CT. Neurophysiological observations in diseased newborns. Biol Psychiatry 1975; 10:527–58.

34. Hagne I. Development of the EEG in normal infants during the first year of life. Acta Paediatr Scand [Suppl] 1972; 232:1–53.

35. Hughes JR, Fino J, Gagnon L. The use of the electroencephalogram in the confirmation of seizures in premature and neonatal infants. Neuropaediatrie 1983; 14:213–9.
36. Clancy RR. Interictal sharp EEG transients in neonatal seizures. J Child Neurol 1989; 4:30–38.
37. Rose AL, Lombroso CT. Neonatal seizure states. A study of clinical, pathological and EEG features in 137 full term babies with long-term follow-up. Pediatrics 1970; 45:404–25.
38. Kellaway P, Crawley J. A primer of electroencephalography of infants. Sections I and II. Methodology and criteria of normality. Bethesda: NIH, 1964.
39. Tharp BR. Neonatal electroencephalography. In: Korobkin R, Guilleminault C, eds. Progress in perinatal neurology. Baltimore: Williams and Wilkins, 1981; 31–64.
40. Dreyfus-Brisac C, Monod N. The electroencephalogram of full-term new-born and premature infants. In: Lairy GC, ed. Handbook of electroencephalography and clinical neurophysiology. Amsterdam: Elsevier, 1975; 6:6–24.
41. Parmelee AH, Stern E. Development of states in infants. In: Clemente CD, Purpura DP, Mayer F, eds. Sleep and the maturing nervous system. New York: Academic, 1972; 199–228.
42. Ellingson RJ. Cortical electrical responses to visual stimulation in the human infant. Electroencephalogr Clin Neurophysiol 1960; 12:663–77.
43. Weitzman ED, Graziani LJ. Maturation and topography of the auditory evoked response of prematurely born infant. Dev Psychobiol 1968; 1:79–89.
44. Petersén I, Eeg-Olofsson O. The development of the electroencephalogram in normal children from the age of 1 through 15 years—non-paroxysmal activity. Neuropaediatrie 1971; 2:247–304.
45. Schoppenhorst M, Brauer F, Freund G, Kubicki S. The significance of coherence estimates in determining central alpha and mu activities. Electroencephalogr Clin Neurophysiol 1980; 48:25–33.
46. Niedermeyer E. The generalized epilepsies. Springfield, Ill.: C. C. Thomas, 1972; 247.
47. Magnus O. The central alpha-rhythm ("rythme en arceau"). Electroencephalogr Clin Neurophysiol 1954; 6:349–50.
48. Bogart KC, Smith DL. Clinical correlates of unilateral mu. Clin EEG, 1978; 9:181–85.
49. Ellingson, RJ. EEGs of premature and full-term newborns. In: Klass, DW, Daly, DD, eds. Current practice of clinical electroencephalography. New York: Raven, 1979; 149–77.
50. Millichap JG, Madsen JA, Aledort LM. Studies in febrile seizures. V. Clinical and electroencephalographic study in unselected patients. Neurology (Minneap) 1960; 10:643–53.
51. Metcalf DR, Jordan K. EEG ontogenesis in normal children. In: Smith WL, ed. Drugs, development and cerebral function. Springfield, Ill.: C. C. Thomas, 1972.
52. Metcalf DR, Mondale J, Butler FK. Ontogenesis of spontaneous K-complexes. Psychophysiology 1971; 8:340–7.
53. Kellaway P, Fox BJ. Electroencephalographic diagnosis of cerebral pathology in infants during sleep. I. Rationale, technique and the characteristics of normal sleep in infants. J Pediatr 1952, 41:262–87.

54. Werner SS, Stockard JE, Bickford RG. Atlas of neonatal electroencephalography. New York: Raven, 1977; 211.

55. Dreyfus C, Curzi-Dascalova L. The EEG during the first year of life. In: Lairy GC, ed. Handbook of electroencephalography and clinical neurophysiology. Amsterdam: Elsevier, 1975; 6:24–30.

56. Gibbs FA, Gibbs EL. Atlas of electroencephalography. Reading, Mass.: Addison-Wesley, 1950, 1:324.

57. Santamaria J, Chiappa KH. The EEG in drowsiness. New York: Demos, 1987; 202.

58. Vignaendra J, Matthews RL, Chatrian GE. Positive occipital sharp transients of sleep: relationships to nocturnal sleep cycle in man. Electroencephalogr Clin Neurophysiol 1974; 37:239–46.

59. Gutierrez-Luque AG, MacCarty CS, Klass DW. Head injury with suspected subdural hematoma: effect on EEG. Arch Neurol 1966; 15:437–43.

60. Menšiková Z. The nature of the space occupying process. In: Magnus O, ed. Handbook of electroencephalography and clinical neurophysiology. Amsterdam: Elsevier, 1975; 14(C):36–49.

61. Arfel G, Fischgold H. EEG signs in tumours of the brain. Electroencephalogr Clin Neurophysiol 1961; Suppl 19:36–50.

62. Vander Drift JHA, Kok NKD, Niedermeyer E, Naquet R, Vigouroux RA. The EEG in relation to pathology in simple cerebral ischemia. In: Vander Drift, JHA, ed. Handbook of electroencephalography and clinical neurophysiology. Amsterdam: Elsevier, 1972; 13A:17–46.

63. Daly DD. The effect of sleep upon the electroencephalogram in patients with brain tumors. Electroencephalogr Clin Neurophysiol 1968; 25:521–9.

64. Falconer MA, Kennedy WA. Epilepsy due to small focal temporal lesions with bilateral independent spike-discharging foci. J Neurol Neurosurg Psychiatry 1961; 24:205–12.

65. Jung R, Riechert R, Meyer-Mickeleit RW. Über intracerebrale Hirnpotentialableitungen bei hirnchirurgischen Eingriffen. Dtsche Z Nervenheilk 1950; 162:52–60.

66. Fischgold H, Pertuiset B, Arfel-Capdeville G. Quelques particularités électroencéphalographiques au niveau des brèches et des volets neurochirurgicaux. Rev Neurol (Paris) 1952; 86:126– .

67. Saunders MG, Westmoreland BF. The EEG in evaluation of disorders affecting the brain diffusely. In: Klass DW, Daly DD, eds. Current practice of clinical electroencephalography. New York: Raven, 1979; 343–79.

68. Goldensohn ES. Use of the EEG for evaluation of focal intracranial lesions. In: Klass DW, Daly DD, eds. Current practice of clinical electroencephalography. New York: Raven, 1979; 307–41.

69. Chaptal J, Jean R, Campo C, Carli N, Passouant P, Cadilhac J. Étude sur le myxoedème de l'enfant. Arch Fr Pediatr 1956; 13:509–36.

70. Passouant P, Cadilhac J, Jean R. Les anomalies EEG selon l'origine thyroidienne ou cérébrale du myxoedème de l'enfant. Rev neurol 1956; 95:569–71.

71. Cadilhac J. EEG in thyroid dysfunction. In: Glaser GH, ed. Handbook of electroencephalography and clinical neurophysiology. Amsterdam: Elsevier, 1976; 15C:70–76.

72. Oken BS, Kaye JA. Electrophysiologic function in the healthy extremely old. Neurology (Minneap) 1992; 42:519–26.

73. Drachman DA, Hughes JR. Memory and the hippocampal complexes. III. Aging and temporal EEG abnormalities. Neurology (Minneap) 1971; 21:1–14.
74. Gloor P. Generalized and widespread bilateral paroxysmal activities. In: Cobb, WA, ed. Handbook of electroencephalography and clinical neurophysiology. Amsterdam, Elsevier, 1976; 11B:52–87.
75. Eeg-Olofsson O: The development of the electroencephalogram in normal adolescents from the age of 16 through 21 years. Neuropaediatrie 1971; 3: 11–45.
76. Dongier M. Mental diseases. In: Gastaut, H, ed. Handbook of electroencephalography and clinical neurophysiology. Amsterdam: Elsevier, 1974; 13B: 22–59.
77. Hess R. Elektroencephalographische studien bei hirntumoren. Stuttgart: Thieme, 1958; 106.
78. Blackwood W, Corsellis JAN, eds. Greenfield's neuropathology. Chicago: Year Book, 1976.
79. Hughes JR, Cayaffa JJ. The EEG in patients at different ages without organic cerebral disease. Electroencephalogr Clin Neurophysiol 1977; 42:776–84.
80. Maynard SD, Hughes JR. A distinctive electrographic entity: bursts of rhythmical temporal theta. Clin EEG 1984; 15:145–50.
81. Gibbs FA, Gibbs EL. Age factor in epilepsy: a summary and synthesis. N Engl J Med 1963; 269:1230–6.
82. Niedermeyer E. EEG and old age. In: Niedermeyer E, Lopes da Silva F, eds. Electroencephalography. 2nd Ed. Baltimore: Urban & Schwarzenberg, 1987; 301–8.
83. Visser SL, Hooijer C, Jonker C, Van Tilburg W, DeRijke W. Anterior temporal focal abnormalities in EEG in normal aged subjects: correlations with psychological and CT brain scan findings. Electroencephalogr Clin Neurophysiol 1987; 66:1–7.
84. Hughes JR. A statistical analysis on the location of EEG abnormalities. Electroencephalogr Clin Neurophysiol 1960; 12:905–9.
85. Courville CB. Traumatic lesions of the temporal lobe as the essential cause of psychomotor epilepsy. In: Baldwin M, Bailey P, eds. Temporal lobe epilepsy. Springfield, Ill.: Thomas, 1958; 220–39.
86. Cobb WA, Müller G. Parietal focal theta rhythm. Electroencephalogr Clin Neurophysiol 1954; 6:455–60.
87. Decker DA Jr, Knott JR. The EEG in intrinsic supratentorial brain tumors: a comparative evaluation. Electroencephalogr Clin Neurophysiol 1972; 33: 303–10.
88. Doose H, Gundel A. 4 to 7 CPS rhythm in childhood EEG. In: Anderson VE, Hauser WA, Penry JK, Sing CF, eds. Genetic basis of the epilepsies. New York: Raven, 1982; 83–93.
89. Aird RB, Gastaut Y. Occipital and posterior electroencephalographic rhythms. Electroencephalogr Clin Neurophysiol 1959; 11:637–56.
90. Martinius J, Matthes A, Lombroso CT. Electroencephalographic features in posterior fossa tumors in children. Electroencephalogr Clin Neurophysiol 1968; 25:128–39.
91. Mizuno Y, Hughes JR. EEG in transient ischemic attacks. Dis Nerv Syst 1972; 33:126–35.
92. Pollen DA. Intracellular studies of cortical neurons during thalamic induced wave and spike. Electroencephalogr Clin Neurophysiol 1964; 17:398–404.

93. Ajmone-Marsan C. Depth electrography and electrocorticography. In: Aminoff MJ, ed. Electrodiagnosis in clinical neurology. New York: Churchill Livingstone, 1980; 167–96.

94. Gibbs FA, Gibbs EL. Atlas of electroencephalography. Vol. 2 Epilepsy. Reading, Mass.: Addison-Wesley, 1952.

95. Lairy GC, Harrison A. Functional aspects of EEG foci in children—clinical data and longitudinal studies. In: Kellaway P, Petersén I, eds. Clinical electroencephalography in children. Stockholm: Almquist and Wiksell, 1968.

96. Cavazzuti GB, Cappella L, Nalin A. Longitudinal study of epileptiform EEG patterns in normal children. Epilepsia 1980; 21:43–55.

97. Hughes JR. The significance of the interictal spike discharge: a review. J Clin Neurophysiol 1989; 6(3):207–26.

98. Shewmon DA, Erwin RJ. The effect of focal interictal spikes on perception and reaction time. General considerations. Electroencephalogr Clin Neurophysiol. 1988; 69:319–37.

99. Kasteleijn-Nolst Trenite DGA, Riemersma JBJ, Binnie CD, Smit AM, Meinarde H. The influence of subclinical epileptiform EEG discharge in driving behavior. Electroencephalogr Clin Neurophysiol 1987; 67:167–70.

100. Morrell F. Physiology and histochemistry of the mirror focus. In: Jasper HH, Ward AA, Pope A, eds. Basic mechanisms of the epilepsies. Boston: Little, Brown, 1969; 357–70.

101. Hughes JR. Long-term clinical and EEG change in patients with epilepsy. Arch Neurol 1985; 42:213–23.

102. Trojaborg W. Focal spike discharges in children, a longitudinal study. Acta Paediatr Scand [Suppl 168] 1966; 55:1–13.

103. Katsurada M. L'électroencéphalogramme de 28 infants nés a term. décédés avant un an. Essai d'interprétation. Fac Méd (Paris) 1967; 24.

104. Dreyfus-Brisac C, Monod N. Sleeping behavior in abnormal newborn infants. Neuropaediatrie 1970; 1:354–66.

105. Cukier F, Andre M, Monod N, Dreyfus-Brisac C. Apport de l'EEG au diagnostic des hémorragies intra-ventriculaires du prématuré. Rev. Electroencephalogr Neurophysiol Clin 1972; 2:318.

106. Monod N, Dreyfus-Brisac C, Sfaello Z. Depistage et pronostic de l'état de mal neonatal d'après électroclinique de 150 cas. Arch Fr Pediatr 1969; 26:1085–102.

107. Hughes JR, Kuhlman DT, Hughes CA. Electro-clinical correlations of positive and negative sharp waves on the temporal and central areas in premature infants. Clin EEG 1991; 22(1):30–9.

108. Chung HJ, Clancy RR. Significance of positive temporal sharp waves in the neonatal electroencephalogram. Electroencephalogr Clin Neurophysiol 1991; 79(4):256–63.

109. Kellaway P, Mizrahi EM. Clinical, electroencephalographic, therapeutic and pathophysiologic studies of neonatal seizures. In: Wasterlain CG, Vert P, eds. Neonatal seizures. New York: Raven, 1990; 1–14.

110. Passouant P, Cadilhac J. EEG and clinical study of epilepsy during maturation in man. Epilepsia 1962; 3:14–43.

111. Plouin P. Benign neonatal convulsions, In: Wasterlain CG, Vert P, eds. Neonatal seizures. New York: Raven, 1990; 51–9.

112. Goldberg HJ, Sheehy EM. Fifth day fits: an acute zinc deficiency syndrome? Arch Dis Child 1983; 57:633–5.

113. Ohtahara S. Seizure disorders in infancy and childhood. Brain Dev 1984; 6:509–19.
114. Aicardi J. Neonatal myoclonic encephalopathy and early infantile epileptic encephalopathy. In: Wasterlain CG, Vert P, eds. Neonatal seizures. New York: Raven, 1990, pp. 41–9.
115. Bickford RG, Klass DW. Scalp and depth electrographic studies of electrodecremental seizures. Electroencephalogr Clin Neurophysiol 1960; 12:263.
116. Sorel L, Dusaucy-Bauloye A. A propos de 21 cas d'hypsarythmie de Gibbs. Son traitement spectaculaire par l'ACTH. Acta Neurol Belg 1958; 58:130–41.
117. Glaser GH. Mechanisms of antiepileptic drug action: clinical indicators. In: Glaser GH, Penry JK, Woodbury DM, eds. Antiepileptic drugs: mechanisms of action. New York: Raven, 1980; 11–20.
118. Commission on Classification and Terminology of the ILAE Proposal for Revised Classification of Epilepsies and Epileptic Syndromes. Epilepsia 1989; 30:389–99.
119. West WJ. On a peculiar form of infantile convulsion. Lancet 1841; 1:724–5.
120. Lennox W, Lennox MA. Epilepsy and related disorders. Vols. I and II. London: Churchill, 1960, 1168 pp.
121. Gastaut H, Roger J, Souloyrol R, Tassinari CA, Régis H, Dravet C, Bernard R, Pinsard N, Saint-Jean M. Childhood epileptic encephalopathy with diffuse slow spike-waves otherwise known as "petit mal variant" or Lennox syndrome. Epilepsia 1966; 7:139–79.
122. Gastaut H, Roger J, Ouachi S, Timsit M, Broughton R. An electroclinical study of generalized epileptic seizures of tonic expression. Epilepsia 1963; 4:15–44.
123. Oller-Daurella L. The EEG and the treatment of epilepsy. In: Gastaut H, ed. Handbook of electroencephalography and clinical neurophysiology. Amsterdam: Elsevier, 1975, 13A:87–91.
124. Gastaut H, Low MD. Antiepileptic properties of clobazam, a 1,5 benzodiazepine. Epilepsia 1971; 12:197–214.
125. The Felbamate Study Group in Lennox-Gastaut Syndrome. Efficacy of felbamate in childhood epileptic encephalopathy (Lennox-Gastaut Syndrome.) N Engl J Med 1993; 328:29–33.
126. Browne TR, Penry JK, Porter RJ, Dreifuss FE. Responsiveness before, during and after spike-wave paroxysms. Neurology (Minneap) 1974; 24:659–65.
127. Penfield W, Jasper H. Epilepsy and the functional anatomy of the human brain. Boston: Little, Brown, 1954.
128. Gloor P. Generalized cortico-reticular epilepsies: some considerations on the pathophysiology of generalized bilaterally synchronus spike-and-slow wave discharge. Epilepsia 1968; 9:249–63.
129. Daly DD. Use of the EEG for diagnosis and evaluation of epileptic seizures and nonepileptic episodic disorders. In: Klass DW, Daly DD, eds. Current practice of clinical electroencephalography. New York: Raven, 1979; 221–68.
130. Niedermeyer E. The generalized epilepsies. Springfield, Ill.: Thomas, 1972.
131. Metrakos K, Metrakos JD. Genetics of convulsive disorders. II. Genetic and electroencephalographic studies in centrencephalic epilepsy. Neurology (Minneap) 1961; 11:474–83.
132. Degen R, Degen HE, Roth CH. Some genetic aspects of idiopathic and symptomatic absence seizures: waking and sleep EEGs in siblings. Epilepsia 1990; 31(6):784–94.

133. Ferrendelli JA, Kupferberg HJ. Antiepileptic drugs. Succinimides. In: Glaser GH, Penry JK, Woodbury DM, eds. Antiepileptic drugs: mechanisms of action. New York: Raven, 1980; 587–96.
134. Snead OC, Hosey LC. Exacerbation of seizures in children by carbamazepine. N Engl J Med 1985; 313:916–21.
135. Lance JW, Anthony M. Sodium valproate and clonazepam in the treatment of intractable epilepsy. Arch Neurol 1977; 34:14–17.
136. Gibbs EL, Fois A, Gibbs FA. The electroencephalogram in retrolental fibroplasia. New Engl J Med 1955; 253:1102–6.
137. Ludwig BI, Ajmone-Marsan C. Clinical ictal patterns in epileptic patients with occipital electroencephalographic foci. Neurology (Minneap) 1975; 25:463–71.
138. Gastaut H. A new type of epilepsy: benign partial epilepsy of childhood with occipital spike-waves. Clin EEG 1982; 13:13–22.
139. Bancaud J, Colomb D, Dell MB. Les pointes rolandiques: un symptôme. E.E.G. propre a l'enfant. Rev Neurol 1958; 99:206–9.
140. Beaussart M, Faou R. Evolution of epilepsy with rolandic paroxysmal foci: a study of 324 cases. Epilepsia 1978; 19:337–42.
141. Bray P, Wiser W. Evidence for a genetic etiology of temporal-central abnormalities in focal epilepsy. N. Engl J Med 1964; 271:926–33.
142. Lerman P, Livity S. Benign focal epilepsy of childhood. A follow-up study of 100 recovered patients. Arch Neurol 1975; 32:261–4.
143. Nayrac P, Beaussart M. Les pointes-ondes prérolandiques. Expression EEG très particulière. Étude électroclinique de 21 cas. Rev Neurol 1958; 99: 201–206.
144. Legarda S, Jayakar P, Alvarez L, Resnick T, Duchowny M. Benign rolandic epilepsy: high central and low central subgroups. Proc Amer EEG Soc 1992, 55.
145. DeMarco P. The benign infantile epilepsies with evoked spikes. Clin EEG 1985; 16(1):39–44.
146. Tharp BR. Orbital frontal seizures. A unique electroencephalographic and clinical syndrome. Epilepsia 1972; 13:627–42.
147. Talwar D, Rask CA, Torres F. Clinical manifestations in children with occipital spike-wave paroxysms. Epilepsia 1992; 33(4):667–74.
148. Tassinari CA, Bureau M, Dravet C, Roger J, Danile Natale O. Electrical status epilepticus during sleep in children (ESES). In: Sterman MB, Shouse MN, Passouant P, eds. Electroencephalography. 2nd ed. Baltimore: Urban & Schwarzenberg, 1987; 405–510.
149. Hughes JR, Olson SF. An investigation of eight different types of temporal lobe discharges. Epilepsia 1981; 22:421–35.
150. Pourmand RA, Markand ON, Thomas C. Midline spike discharges: Clinical and EEG correlations. Clin EEG 1984; 15:232–7.
151. Chatrian GE, Shaw CM, Leffman H. The significance of periodic lateralized epileptiform discharges in EEG: an electrographic, clinical and pathological study. Electroencephalogr Clin Neurophysiol 1964; 17:177–93.
152. Hughes JR, Schlagenhauff RE. The periodically recurring focal discharge. Epilepsia 1965; 6:156–66.
153. Grand'Maison F, Reiher J, Leduc CP. Retrospective inventory of EEG abnormalities in partial status epilepicus. Electroencephalogr Clin Neurophysiol 1991; 79:264–70.

154. Markand ON. Electroencephalography in diffuse encephalopathies. J Clin Neurophysiol 1984; 1:357–407.
155. Niedermeyer E. Abnormal EEG patterns (epileptic and paroxysmal). In: Niedermeyer E, Lopes Da Silva F, eds. Electroencephalography, 2nd ed. Baltimore: Urban & Schwarzenberg, 1989; 183–207.
156. Lombroso CT, Schwartz IH, Clark DM, Meunch H, Barry J. Ctenoids in healthy youths: controlled study of 14- and 6-per second positive spiking. Neurology (Minneap) 1966; 16:1152–8.
157. Gibbs EL, Gibbs FA. Electroencephalographic evidence of thalamic and hypothalamic epilepsy. Neurology (Minneap) 1951; 1:136–44.
158. Henry CE. Positive spike discharges in the EEG and behavior abnormality. In: Glaser GH, ed. EEG and behavior. New York: Basic Books, 1963; 315–44.
159. Hughes JR. A review of the positive spike phenomenon. In: Wilson W, ed. Applications of electroencephalography in psychiatry. Durham, N.C.: Duke University Press, 1965; 54–101.
160. Bosaeus E, Sellden U. Psychiatric assessment of healthy children with various EEG patterns. Acta Psychiatr Scand 1979; 59:180–210.
161. Lipman I, Hughes JR. Rhythmic mid-temporal discharges. An electroclinical study. Electroencephalogr Clin Neurophysiol 1969; 27:43.
162. Boutros NN, Hughes JR, Weiler M. Psychiatric correlates of rhythmic mid temporal discharges and 6/sec spike and wave complexes. Biol Psychiatr 1986; 21:94–9.
163. Hughes JR, Hermann BP. Evidence for psychopathology in patients with rhythmic midtemporal discharges. Biol Psychiatr 1984; 19(12):1623–34.
164. Hughes JR, Cayaffa JJ. Is the "psychomotor variant" "rhythmic mid temporal discharge" an ictal pattern? Clin EEG 1973; 4:42–9.
165. Hughes JR. Two forms of the 6/sec spike and wave complex. Electroencephalogr Clin Neurophysiol 1980; 48:535–50.
166. Hughes JR, Fino JJ. Changes in reactivity during the 6/second spike and wave complex. Clin EEG 1992; 23(1):31–6.
167. Reiher J, Klass DW. Two common EEG patterns of doubtful clinical significance. Med Clin North Am 1968; 52:933–40.
168. White J, Langston W, Pedley T. Benign epileptiform transients of sleep. Neurology (Minneap) 1977; 27:1061–8.
169. Koshino Y, Niedermeyer E. The clinical significance of small sharp spikes in the electroencephalogram. Clin EEG 1975; 6:131–40.
170. Hughes JR, Gruener G. Small sharp spikes revisited: further data on this controversial pattern. Clin EEG 1984; 15:208–13.
171. Molaie M, Santana DB, Otero C, Cavanaugh WA. Effect of epilepsy and sleep deprivation on the rate of benign epileptiform transients of sleep. Epilepsia 1991; 32(1):44–50.
172. Reiher J, Lebel M. Wicket spikes: clinical correlates of a previously undescribed EEG pattern. Can J Neurol Sci 1977; 4:39–47.
173. Bickford RG, Butts HR. Hepatic coma: the electroencephalographic pattern. J Clin Invest 1955; 34:790–9.
174. Mahurkar SD, Dhar SK, Salta R, Meyers L, Smith EC, Dunea G. Dialysis dementia. Lancet 1973; 1:1412–5.
175. Foley JM, Watson CW, Adams RD. Significance of the electroencephalographic changes in hepatic coma. Trans Am Neurol Assoc 1950; 75:161–5.

176. Silverman D. Some observations on the EEG in hepatic coma. Electroenceph-alogr Clin Neurophysiol 1962; 14:53–9.
177. Cobb W. The periodic events of subacute sclerosing leucoencephalitis. Electroencephalogr Clin Neurophysiol 1966; 21:278–94.
178. Johnson LC, Seales DM, Naitoh P, Church MW, Sinclair M. The effects of flurazepam hydrochloride on brain electrical activity. Electroencephalogr Clin Neurophysiol 1979; 47:309–21.
179. White J, Tharp B. An arousal pattern in children with organic cerebral dysfunction. Electroencephalogr Clin Neurophysiol 1974; 37:265–8.
180. Morse HN. The aberrational man—a tour de force of legal psychiatry. J Forensic Sci 1968; 13:1–13, 365–9, 488–97.
181. Woolsey RM, Goldner JA. Forensic aspects of electroencephalography. Med Trial Tech 1975; Winter:338–48.
182. Gibbs FA, Gibbs EL. Atlas of Electroencephalography. Vol. 3. Cambridge, Mass.: Addison-Wesley, 1964; 538 pp.
183. Gibbs FA, Weigner WR, Gibbs EL. The electroencephalogram in post-traumatic epilepsy. Am J Psychiatry 1944; 100:738–49.
184. Courjon J. Handbook of electroencephalography and clinical neurophysiology. Vol. 14 Part B. Traumatic disorders. 1972; 104 pp.
185. Jung R. Neurophysiologische Untersuchungsmethoden. In: Von Bergmann G et al., (Herausg.) Handbuch der inneren medizin. Berlin: Springer; Heidelberg: Göttingen, 1953; 1:1206–420.
186. Götze W, Wolter M. Grenzen der hirnstromuntersuchung bei der begutachtung von hirntraumafolgen. Med sachverst 1957; 53:104–9.
187. Williams D. The electroencephalogram in chronic post-traumatic states. J Neurol Psychiatry 1941; 4:131–46.
188. Marshall C, Walker AE. The value of electroencephalography in the prognostication and prognosis of post-traumatic epilepsy. Epilepsia (Amst) 1961; 2:138–43.
189. Courjon J. Apport de l'exploration fonctionelle du système nerveux dans le diagnostic et le pronostic des traumatismes crâniens récents. Acta Neurol Belg 1970; 70:359–77.
190. Gibbs FA, Gibbs EL. Atlas of electroencephalography. Vol. 2. Cambridge, Mass.: Addison-Wesley, 1952; 422 pp.
191. Planques J, Grèzes-Rueff CH. L'électroencéphalographic dans l'expertise médico-légale. XXVIIeme Congres International de Médecine du Travail. Médecine Legale et Médecine Sociale de Langue Francaise. Imp. A. Coueslant. Strasbourg: Cahors, 1954; 309.
192. Meyer-Mickeleit RW. Das Electroencephalogram nach gedeckten kopfverletzungen. Dtsch Med Wschr 1953; 1:480–4.
193. Scherzer E. Über die gutachtliche Wertung des 4/sec. Rhythmus nach Schadeltraumen. Psychiatr et Neurol (Basel) 1965; 150:8–20.
194. Vogel F. Genetiche Aspekte des Electroencephalograms. Sich Med Wschr 1963; 88:1748–59.
195. Belli MM. Modern trials. Indianapolis: Bobbs-Merrill, 1954; 569 pp.
196. Phillips, G. Traumatic epilepsy after closed head injury. J Neurol Neurosurg 1954; 17:1–10.
197. Jasper H, Penfield W. Electroencephalograms in post-traumatic epilepsy. Am J Psychiatry 1943; 100:365–77.

198. Jennett B. Epilepsy after non-missile head injuries. London: Heinemann, 1975; 179 pp.

199. Ascroft PB. Traumatic epilepsy after gunshot wounds of the head. Br Med J 1941; 1:739–44.

200. Perr IN. Medico-legal aspects of post-traumatic epilepsy. Am J Psychiatry 1960; 116:981–92.

201. Hyslop GH. Seizures, head injuries and litigants. Indust Hyg Toxicol 1949; 31:336–42.

202. Silverman D. Clinical and electroencephalographic studies on criminal psychopaths. Arch Neurol Psychiatry 1943; 50:18–33.

203. Gibbs FA, Bloomberg W, Bagchi BK. Electroencephalographic study of criminals. Am J Psychiatry 1945; 102:294–8.

204. Kennard MA, Rabinovitch MS, Fister WP. The use of frequency analysis in the interpretation of EEGs of patients with psychological disorders. Electroencephalogr Clin Neurophysiol 1955; 7:29–38.

205. Hill D, Pond DA. Reflections on one hundred capital cases submitted to electroencephalography. J Ment Sci 1952; 98:23–43.

206. Hill D. EEG in episodic, psychotic and psychopathic behavior. A classification of date. Electroencephalogr Clin Neurophysiol 1952; 4:419–42.

207. Winkler GE, Kove SS. Implications of electroencephalographic abnormalities in homicide cases. Neuropsychiatry 1962; 3:322–30.

208. Levy S, Kennard MA. Study of electroencephalogram as related to personality structure in group of inmates of state penitentiary. Am J Psychiatry 1953; 109:82–9.

209. Small JE. The organic dimension of crime. Arch Gen Psychiatry 1966; 15:82–9.

210. Stafford-Clark D, Taylor FH. Clinical and electroencephalographic studies of prisoners charged with murder. J Neurosurg Psychiatry 1949; 12:325–30.

211. Stafford-Clark D, Pond D, Doust JWL. The psychopath in prison: a preliminary report of a co-operative research. Br J Delinq 1951; 2:117.

212. Silverman D. The electroencephalogram of criminals. Arch Neurol Psychiatry 1944; 52:38–42.

213. Williams D. Neural factors related to habitual aggression: considerations of differences between those habitual aggressors and others who have committed crimes of violence. Brain 1969; 92:503–20.

214. Levy S. A study of the electroencephalogram as related to personality structure in a group of inmates of a state penitentiary. Electroencephalogr Clin Neurophysiol 1952; 4:113.

215. Alström CH. A study of epilepsy in its clinical, social, and genetic aspects. Copenhagen: Ejnar Munksgaard, 1950; 284 pp.

216. Mark VH, Ervin FR. Violence and the brain. New York: Harper and Row, 1970; 170 pp.

217. Walton JN. Some observations on the value of electroencephalography in medico-legal practice. Medicoleg J 1963; 31:15–35.

218. Curran D. Psychiatry Ltd. J Ment Sci 1952; 98–373.

219. Southern EEG Society. Electroencephalography and the law. Moot trial proceedings on two cases. Birmingham, Ala., Oct. 26, 1968.

220. Lennox WG. Epilepsy and related disorders. Boston: Little, Brown, 1960; 2:965–94.

221. Delgado-Escueta AV, Mattson RH, King L, Goldensohn ES, Spiegel H, Madsen J, Crandall P, Dreifuss F, Porter RJ. The nature of aggression during epileptic seizures. N Engl J Med 1981; 305:711–6.
222. Kiloh LG, Osselton JW. Clinical electroencephalography. London: Butterworth and Co., 1961; 135 pp.

Index